# A Secret Life

*Enduring and Triumphing Over OCD:*
*Obsessive Compulsive Disorder*

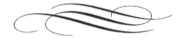

James S. Juliana

A Secret Life
© 2019 James S. Juliana

First Edition

ISBN 978-0-578-52389-7

Edited by Stephen and Joyce Singular
Book layout and design by Gail Nelson, e-book-design.com

Printed in the United States of America

*For Bette; you taught me to love and be empathetic.*

*To Betsy; you are the love of my life and best friend.*

*To our children and grandchildren; thank you for your love and understanding.*

# Table of Contents

# Introduction

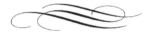

$O$n multiple occasions throughout my teaching career, especially during my early years of teaching in the classroom, I often felt as if I was on an island, isolated from the outside world, while facing the challenging behavior of teenagers. Likewise, my wife Betsy and I have often felt alone when dealing with the multiple pitfalls of my secret life, living with Obsessive Compulsive Disorder. I know there are individuals today confronting this same maddening reality, and I want to speak to them, if not for them. You are not alone.

If you have ever experienced Obsessive Compulsive Disorder symptoms, if your life has been interrupted because of this insidious disorder, if you have a family member or friend who deals daily with a form of obsessive and/or compulsive thoughts and behaviors, I strongly urge you to continue reading.

Four years ago, I read about the saga of two young Colorado women, twin sisters in their early twenties, who had struggled with mental health issues since childhood. In adolescence they were diagnosed with severe OCD. The girls rarely left home for fears related to using public restrooms.

They followed a ritual of repeatedly disinfecting their skin with rubbing alcohol until their flesh burned. They took showers lasting for hours and suffered from severe depression. OCD was controlling their lives.

In 2015, the young women underwent revolutionary surgery to implant electrode wires in their heads, necks and shoulders. The electrodes were attached to a battery pack and inserted in their chests. Their physician electronically controlled their OCD impulses through brain stimulation. Immediately following the surgery, the twins believed they had discovered the solution to their lives having been distorted and overtaken by OCD. Finally, they would be able to live much more normally. After reading the article, I remember hoping against hope this technique would be effective for the sisters.

In April of 2018, the sisters committed suicide together. The medical strategy had obviously failed. Sadness and sorrow overwhelmed me when I said a silent prayer for them. What a waste and loss, I thought, as I questioned my psychologist about the sisters' tragedy at our next appointment. Dr. Gallagher was very aware of the situation, having met the sisters several years earlier while participating in an OCD forum. No life, he assured me, should be cut short because of a mental illness or phobia, yet these two young lives had been taken away by OCD. I understood this scenario from the inside out, because my life could have easily ended many times as a result of my secret life dealing with OCD.

My entire adolescence and adulthood have been intertwined with confronting, overcoming and ultimately defeating the curse of OCD. I consider myself an expert on succeeding in life despite living with OCD—even before physicians understood, defined and could attempt to treat it. Countless times, I have endured severe depression, suicidal thoughts, debilitating anxiety, recurring feelings of lacking self-worth or self-esteem, a proclivity for physical violence, a disdain for authority, the loss of employment and a general malaise regarding my purpose in life.

While also experiencing exhilarating highs and personal successes, I have felt possessed by the devil. Wherever you have visited in your own mind, I have been there or close by. For decades I constantly searched for different medications and more effective therapies to control my OCD, all in vain. Finally, after treatment by a dozen specialists, and after taking so many medications I cannot recall all of their names, my life has recently changed dramatically through the combination of using one drug and participating in one specific therapy.

My wife Betsy and I do not want OCD sufferers to experience the hopelessness and depression I have known and that she has shared with me. Through writing this book, we want readers to discover avenues of hope and relief in their fight against OCD and its symptoms.

### Goals

My life's vocation has been teaching and mentoring children and adolescents to become intelligent, articulate and empathetic adults. Betsy and I trust that this book will also be an educational tool, providing people with the understanding that medical professionals, therapies and medications can significantly assist individuals and their loved ones suffering with OCD. We offer our story so that others might live happier, more productive lives.

## Focus

This book is written for OCD patients, their families and friends; psychologists and psychiatrists; other mental health professionals; graduate students in psychology and anyone else trying to help an OCD sufferer.

*You cannot go back and change the beginning, but you can start where you are and change the ending.*
—C. S. Lewis

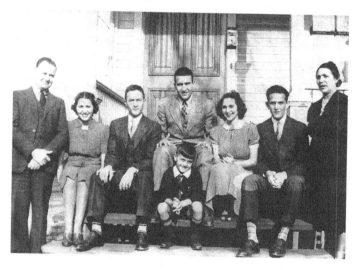

Juliana Family, Circa 1940
Moorestown, N.J.
L-R: Nick, Rae, Jim, Joe, Annetta, Pete, Rose,
and Charles

# Chapter I

# The Mystery

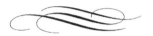

*I* decided to write my story because I have never read a book by someone dealing every day with Obsessive Compulsive Disorder. In medical journals and articles, I have found many quotes and comments from OCD sufferers, but never a full-length work on living with this reality. I grew up with OCD long before it was identified and labeled, and I have battled it since childhood. Endless frustration at not being able to control my obsessions and compulsions has been my lifelong companion and basis for my secret life with OCD.

Instead of another book outlining the causes and variations of OCD, along with the current therapies and medications, I am writing as one who has constantly struggled to overcome OCD. I want to share my journey in the hope my struggles will help others trying to control their own symptoms. In his final book, *The Point of It All*, the extraordinary political commentator and writer Charles Krauthammer wrote that he didn't want his life to be defined by being a quadriplegic confined to a wheelchair, but rather by his achievements. I agree wholeheartedly with Dr. Krauthammer's viewpoint. I want to be defined by what I have accomplished, despite having OCD.

At age 70, I want to attempt to unravel the mystery of this illness and the influences that shaped me. They start with my mother and father; the environment in which I was raised; my faith and its teachings, rules and regulations; my personal values; and finally, my life-long phobia defined as OCD. One core piece of this mystery for me is how I have reached this age without killing myself. And how have I been able to live a meaningful and productive life, while contending with my nemesis?

On December 29, 1948, I was born in St. Vincent's Hospital in mid-town Manhattan, delivered with a rather large, round head, a wide smile, deep brown eyes, and a head full of chocolate brown hair. I was the first of eight children, all boys except for one, born to Jim and Bette Juliana, of Moorestown, New Jersey, a well-to-do Quaker community just across the Delaware River from Philadelphia.

When I arrived, my father had been a Special Agent with the FBI for two years, his primary work being in counter surveillance and intelligence. Jim, or Big Jim as I called him throughout his latter life, infiltrated Communist groups and gathered evidence against those actively attempting to subvert the United States government. Jim was the fifth of six children born to Nicholas and Rose Juliana. His father, Nick, had grown up in South Philly, the son of extremely poor Italian immigrants from Naples, Italy. Nick ended his education before high school and became a vegetable and fruit picker in the fertile truck farms of south Jersey, gathering tomatoes, peppers, lettuce, apples and other fruits and vegetables. At age seven, Rose had immigrated to Philadelphia with her family, who came from a farming village several hours south of Rome, named Potenza.

"Nana" and "Pop" Juliana met as teenage pickers in the Jersey fields, where both families lived in shanties in the summer months. Following marriage, they moved to the tenements of South Philadelphia. Nick secured a well-paying job at Campbell Soup Company in Camden, N.J. and Rose and Nick began raising their large Catholic family. The Juliana family and various close relatives eventually settled in Moorestown, N.J. Nick also worked as a part-time gardener and groundskeeper for local Quakers, while Rose kept house and cooked for some of these same wealthy families.

Rose never allowed the Italian language to be spoken at home, and my father and his siblings knew little of the mother tongue, except for swear words. Their mother was a strict disciplinarian, who emphasized her Catholic faith, her children's education and assimilating into mainstream American society. The Juliana children made outstanding grades and were often All-State athletes, including the two girls. During the Depression, the boys delivered newspapers and ice; their sisters working in child care, sewing and cooking for others.

My maternal grandparents were Joseph Patrick Sutton and Esther Seaman. Patrick's parents were farmers from County Cork, Ireland, who came to America before the turn of the 20th Century. The Suttons had three daughters: my mother Bette, my godmother Alyce, and Mary, ten years younger than my mom. Grandfather Joseph Patrick was one of Moorestown's most successful house and business painters, a leader in the Catholic Church and a member of the Rotary Club. Grandmother Esther, a small woman in stature like Nana Rose, ran the Sutton family household. Esther lived to be a robust 99 and in my eulogy at her funeral I praised her as a prodigious giver—always providing for others.

I was fortunate to receive the love and respect of all four of my grandparents and did everything I could to hide my OCD from them.

My relationship with my father, from the very beginning, was more complicated—perhaps because I was his first-born child and first-born son, with all the expectations that come with this. Dad was a man of accomplishment and measured everyone against that. At Washington College on Maryland's eastern shore, he earned A's and B's, was President of his Kappa Alpha fraternity for two years, and starred on the football and basketball teams. In January 1944, Dad graduated early, magna cum laude, and proceeded directly to Notre Dame University to study to become a deck officer in the U.S. Naval Reserves. His older brother, Joe, was already a Navy pilot fighting in the Aleutian Campaign in Alaska, and his brother Peter was a naval aviator who had survived the attack on Pearl Harbor. Pete's plane and entire crew later went missing on a patrol mission out of Oahu, Hawaii, and remained MIA until the end of the war, when they were declared killed in action.

My father saw combat at Iwo Jima and Okinawa, and brought his ship home safely in 1946 as a full Lieutenant. Following his discharge, he attended the University of Pennsylvania, taking graduate classes in education and renewing his position as a railroad conductor before entering the FBI.

He married Bette in November, 1947.

My mother was 5'9", a shade taller than my dad and a striking blond with sparkling blue eyes and a terrific figure. A superb dancer, Bette had been the lead majorette in her high school band and was later employed as an executive secretary for a large company in Philly. Between my birth and the birth of my next brother, Bette had a miscarriage and then carried another baby who was stillborn–very traumatic experiences for a woman in her mid-twenties. My youngest brothers of eight were twins, and one brother died from a heart defect when two weeks old. Growing up, I felt much closer to my mother than anyone else. I persevered through my childhood and early adolescence because of Bette's love, empathy toward me and the countless hours she spent talking to me about my fears and trepidation caused by OCD.

My family was a strict Catholic family and practicing my faith fervently, even in grade school, was extremely important to me. I was obsessed with being a model Catholic child and never committing any mortal or grievous sins. I wanted to impress my father with my achievements, as he had impressed others. Second through eighth grade I attended an academically-challenging parochial school, administered and taught by Roman Catholic nuns, the Sisters of Charity. The sisters told their students stories about saints in heaven who had endured terrible mental torments and challenges on earth, before the saints triumphed over their obstacles and died. I am no saint; nor do I even wish to intimate that I possess saintly qualities. My life, even then as a young boy, included many transgressions, but I could not help but wonder why I had to endure such treacherous obsessions and compulsions in my secret life from OCD.

My grades were primarily A's with an occasional B. In eighth grade, I ranked in the top ten students in a co-ed class of 60 and fourth among males. I was an altar boy, serving as an assistant to the priest who performed Catholic Masses—a cherished job. I was also a Patrol Boy, a street crossing guard, the captain and quarterback of the eighth grade football team and a starter in baseball. While babysitting six siblings, I changed diapers and fed my three youngest brothers, one of whom was profoundly handicapped developmentally. During his life, my brother David never spoke or displayed any recognition of my parents or his siblings.

Growing up, I was not at all sexually active and remained a virgin until marriage at 23. I was fifteen before I kissed a girl. Yet sex and mortal sin were my omnipresent obsessions throughout my childhood and adolescence. At ten, I began suffering from repetitive, undesired thoughts (obsessions) and/or behaviors (compulsions); more often than not, the thoughts involved a sexual topic or the fear of committing a mortal sin—or both. The incidents occurred in the middle of any activity at home, in school, socially or while participating in athletic or recreational activities. I usually turned the obsessions into a series of rituals, taking a few moments, several minutes or occasionally hours and days to complete them, so I could continue with my life, fast becoming a secret life. Where did all of this come from and what could I do about it—the mystery and challenge in front of me?

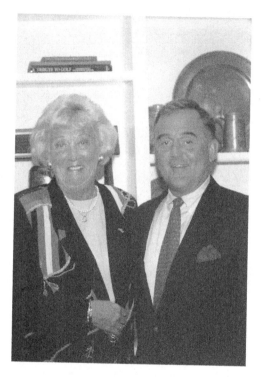

Mother Bette and Author
Bette's 70th birthday, 1973
Atlantic City, N.J.

# Chapter II

# Guilt and Shame

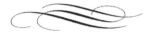

$M$y first OCD incident set off compulsive thoughts so constant and powerful that I lost control of myself. A panel truck was parked in our suburban driveway, belonging to a plumber. It was summer and the weather was warm. While investigating the truck and looking into the cab, I noticed an 8" x 10" colored, detailed drawing of a woman with a naked chest. I was mesmerized and could not take my eyes from the picture.

When I finally turned away, remorse and dread came over me. I immediately experienced intense guilt and worried about having committed a mortal sin. When I went into our house, my mother noticed I was upset and questioned me, but I was reluctant and too embarrassed to answer her.

"What's wrong, sweetheart?" she asked, as I tried to explain the situation to her. "Tell me Jamie—what's the matter? Are you sick? Do you feel okay?"

Her questioning went on for several minutes, as I stood meekly in the kitchen, head bowed, incapable of answering. My stomach had clenched up and I felt flushed and light-headed. How could I tell my mother that I had just repeatedly stared at a picture of a bare-chested woman? A sense of despair overcame me.

After what seemed like forever, I blurted out, "Mom, I just looked at something I should not have looked at. I think I committed a mortal sin. I can't stop thinking about what I saw."

She walked over, took me in her arms, and tightly hugged me.

"Jamie," she said, "you didn't commit a mortal sin. You're too young to do that."

"I looked at a picture of a naked woman. That's a mortal sin."

We tossed the question back and forth, as I became more and more upset.

"A ten year-old cannot commit a mortal sin," she repeated. "God is not going to consider what you did a serious sin. All young boys look at pictures like that. It's just curiosity and that's not a sin."

My mother spent the next hour or more trying to alleviate my feelings and reassuring me that I was not going to hell. I had not, she said again and again, committed a grievous sin against God, because my actions were normal.

After much time and effort on her part and considerable anguish on mine, I was able to consider that perhaps I wasn't dammed to hell for my actions. Maybe, just possibly, she was correct and I had not wanted to commit a mortal sin. The nuns at school had taught me that a person must genuinely have a desire and wish to commit a sin, before an action becomes a mortal sin. With more tears, I embraced my mother and thanked her for helping me realize I was not a grievous sinner. I was physically spent and cannot imagine how Mom must have felt. She had a lot more to deal with than my concerns. As I matured and our family grew, my mother's worries became her own kind of obsession, eventually leading her into alcoholism.

My mother had helped me with this initial incident, but the problem did not go away. This incident initiated an ongoing conflict in my mind throughout my childhood: What actions were or were not mortal, grievous sins? With no knowledge or understanding of OCD, I was beginning my life's journey with this daily burden.

My condition, as I would learn much later, is known as "severe scrupulosity"—thoughts (obsessions) and behaviors (compulsions) dealing with religious guilt—grew through high school. I was developing a very secret, dark, depressing and overwhelming second self, whose actions left me filled with doubt and shame.

At the same time, I was taking on an extraordinary level of responsibility within my family, willing to accept any and all tasks requested of me. No one I knew my age changed as many diapers for his siblings or bathed and dressed them as much as I did. By twelve or thirteen, I was an accomplished babysitter and surrogate parent for six siblings. At school and socially, I was a leader, liked and respected by teachers, coaches and peers. Yet I was shy and reticent around girls and people with authority. I was also uncharacteristically devout and religious. Every May, the month that Catholics devote to the Virgin Mary the Mother of Jesus, I set up a small shrine on my brother's bureau in our bedroom, consisting of a large statue of Mary, arranged with candles and fresh flowers. I considered myself very close to God and Mary then, despite having a dark side. Serving as an altar boy at Mass filled me with contentment, and as an adult, I would become a communion minister. In those situations, I felt at peace with myself, and thought about becoming a Catholic priest.

In sixth grade, while studying Latin responses to become an altar boy, the priest in charge of the altar servers accused me of breaking the rules and cheating on my memorization of my verbal responses. I was devastated by his public allegations, but did not know how to confront him. My dad stepped in and corrected the situation, and I became an altar boy, but remained angry at the priest for questioning my honesty. Never before had anyone in authority reprimanded me for a breech in my value system. I was stunned, especially because the reprimand came from a Catholic priest, the ultimate authority in my young life on matters of good and evil, sin or no sin. This was my introduction to the whims of people with power over me. My concept of moral authority had been challenged by an immature, imperfect young priest, and I felt that my sincere trust had been betrayed. The truth is this feeling has never completely left me.

When trying to manage my OCD symptoms, I often asked myself how a merciful, loving God could allow a ten year-old boy, a caring adolescent and then adult, be controlled by sexual obsessions and compulsions to such an extreme, that I sometimes believed I was possessed by the devil. What I have lived with for six decades is so perverse and outlandish that it is beyond the scope of many horror movies—because this horror is real and intermingled with my close relationship with God.

When I was thirteen or fourteen, a classmate was hit in the head with a baseball and reported to be near death. I rode my bike to church and knelt before the altar, praying as dutifully as I had ever prayed, asking Jesus to spare my friend Vince and allow him to survive and be healthy again. Tears fell down my cheeks and when Vince recovered completely not long afterwards, I experienced a heartfelt belief that my prayers had actually played a very, very small but positive role in Vince being cured.

Around this time, I chose my Uncle Peter, my father's older brother, who was killed on a flying patrol mission in WWII, as my guardian angel and special envoy. In difficult situations or when feeling overwhelmed, I would seek his council and direct prayers to Pete, asking for help and guidance. Today, I still think of his sacrifice when standing for the national anthem at sporting events, and I still pray to him. Some years ago, I wrote a book outlining Peter's military career and attempted to solve the mystery of his final mission. As much as I prayed to God and to Peter, neither seemed able to help me where I needed the most assistance—with my OCD. I was searching for something else that would take decades to find.

As a result of my growing difficulties, I frequently wanted to be alone, reading or building ship and airplane models. I felt safe with them, away from anyone, where no one could observe my obsessions and compulsions.

My secret life was deepening.

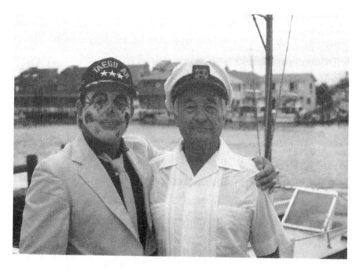

Author and Father Big Jim
Annual Night in Venice Celebration
Ocean City, N.J.

# Chapter III

# Big Jim's Way

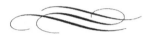

*L*ooking at the photo of the naked lady and feeling extreme guilt was the first time I wondered if something was psychologically and emotionally wrong with me. Then I began having far more disturbing thoughts about women being tortured and having their sexual organs butchered during wartime. I was ten or eleven and must have either watched a movie or program on World War II or read about such atrocities in a war-era book. At that age, I was a voracious reader with an interest in both the Pacific and European Theaters of WWII. I might have read about the terrible tortures in the Nazi concentration camps or the American wars in the west against Native Americans. These thoughts kept surfacing in my mind and now I believed I was most definitely committing mortal sins, but how could I ever talk to my mother about this? As my fear of committing sins grew so did my anger and isolation.

The OCD symptoms and incidents intensified, leaving me with more and more questions: "Why do I have these thoughts and compulsions? Where in the world do they come from? Why me? What is wrong with me?"

Even though I could not tell my mother about this, she

was a constant source of love and solace. My father, as I have said, was another story. When I was young, to me he was superman. I have photos of the two of us when I was three or four, standing together in our bathing suits in the surf at the Jersey shore, and on a dock jutting out into a magnificent lake in the White Mountains of New Hampshire. As I became older, our relationship evolved and became much more entangled. Big Jim was a tough son-of-a-bitch, to put it nicely. If you have ever watched the film *The Great Santini* with Robert Duval as a U.S. Marine aviator, that officer paralleled my father—FBI Special Agent, Chief Council of a Permanent Subcommittee in the United States Senate, friend and confidant of three future US Presidents, and all of this accomplished before 35 years of age. Yet I believe that he, like me, was also an OCD sufferer decades before the phobia was identified or diagnosed. There is reason to believe that the OCD gene was inherited from the Juliana side of the family—according to my father's youngest brother, Charles, my favorite uncle, who confided this to me.

My father's OCD was different from my own. I demanded perfection from myself, while Dad absolutely insisted that his children had to be perfectly behaved, perfectly dressed and perfectly in line with our schoolwork. Every Saturday morning, the older children had a list of chores to do before any sports or fun activities were pursued: rake the leaves, cut the grass, wash the cars, clean the basement, and clean the garage and on and on. Dad created work just to keep us working, with his constant emphasis on cleanliness, organization and even more perfection. As a young boy, I found this excessive—work was a sort of punishment.

When I was a teenager, my mother began to drink heavily. My handicapped brother, David, was placed in a home at age three, and four years later was transferred to a state institution for the developmentally disabled in Woodbine, N.J. Dad and Mother maintained their legal residence in New Jersey, not only because they were originally from the state, but also so our brother David could become a legal resident of the Woodbine Center for the Developmentally Disabled. Senator Robert F. Kennedy, a former co-worker and associate of my father, and his wife Ethel, had recommended Woodbine to my parents during my parents' lengthy and comprehensive search for a residence for David, who was profoundly retarded. So our family spent June through August at the Jersey shore, but Dad rarely was there for more than long weekends, so my mother had ample opportunity to imbibe while Dad was working his job in D.C. By the time I entered high school, Mom was drinking too much and Dad had become her greatest enabler, not taking any steps to curb her disease. Two of my brothers grew up to be alcoholics; one brother has remained sober for many years. I believe that my father shoulders some of the responsibility for that alcoholism as well.

Dad and I had numerous, contentious arguments about stopping mother's drinking. Early on in Mom's drinking, I had spoken with a doctor about this, and all of my siblings agreed to confront our mother about the issue. Dad prevented the intervention, lacking the courage to go along with the plan. He drove us all crazy with his obsessions, his control over us and my mother, his emphasis on perfection in every aspect of our lives, yet he refused to help Mom triumph over her addiction to alcohol. At that point, I began losing faith in my father. He could fight in WWII, be an effective FBI agent, work closely with multiple Presidents of the United States, but could not assist my mother, his wife, when she required it—just as he wasn't compassionate and empathetic with his children. OCD can harm the finest human beings if left untreated. My father never once asked me about my struggles with OCD or talked with me about his own suffering.

In fairness I also remember some good times with my dad. Once in a while, under the right circumstances, Big Jim dropped the military disciplinarian façade and became relaxed and personable, usually after a couple of cocktails at his beach home in south Jersey. Dad was immensely proud of his Ocean City residence, built on a lagoon leading into Great Egg Harbor Bay, just south of Atlantic City. Owning a home on the water and a motorboat were dreams of my father that had come true through dedication and much hard work! Unwinding by the shore, he would say that his most memorable and favorite moments had come in the western Pacific during WWII, as a deck officer on a U.S. Navy warship.

"Jim," he'd tell me, "I loved being on the bridge of the ship and using the stars to navigate our course. Without all the bloodshed, being a naval officer was a beautiful life."

On our large wooden dock, sitting with his younger brother Charles, two of his sons, and the neighborhood baker, Ezio, who happened to be ex-Mafiosa, my father waxed poetic on his work investigating for Senator John F. Kennedy to uncover potential pitfalls prior to his run for the presidency; or Dad's running an FBI probe into New York City's superintendent of public schools and helping her become a government informant and return to the Catholic faith; or receiving a call from the Nixon Administration about constructing a plan for heightened White House security. Dad told many stories of intrigue, undercover assignments and rubbing shoulders with famous individuals. As he smoked cigars and sipped Sambuca, we listened to his tales of travel and accomplishment into the wee hours of the morning. If only he had been able to use his talents or influence and connections to help me in some way with my OCD. In truth, in those years nobody knew what the hell was wrong with me. My fate and my secrets were in Betsy's hands and mine, and we would weather the mental and emotional storms of the future, virtually alone, on a different kind of island, a very secret island.

As my OCD intensified as an adolescent, I began to hurt my siblings on purpose, with an extra shove here, a punch or pinch there. Sitting on the milking stool in our recreation room and watching TV, I would put one of my brother's heads under the stool and force him to lie there perfectly still until I felt like releasing him. When babysitting, I bullied my brothers with physical force if they did not obey me, scaring the hell out of them. Wrestling with them, I used my size and strength to pin them to the carpet and sit on them, but only my brothers. The unwritten rule was that you did not hurt or frighten your sister for fear of severe punishment—getting your buttocks smacked with a hard, flat object. As a "responsible oldest child," I could not let my parents know I was doing any of these things, so my life became even more secretive. If my mother happened to find out about misbehavior, she would say, "Wait until your father gets home." Or, "I can't wait until your father sees that," after I had damaged a piece of furniture or had broken a tool. Awaiting Dad's return, I became sick to my stomach.

For several years in grade school, I was a Cub Scout. I once attended a monthly meeting at another scout's home and became upset over something. I left early and then quit the organization. As an adult, I have repeated this pattern many times—joining a group, feeling disenchanted after encountering an obstacle or being reprimanded, before suddenly bolting for good.

In seventh and eighth grade, I was one of the two or three best athletes in a school of around 500. I disliked basketball because I couldn't hit anyone legally, which is what I most enjoyed. One Saturday we were playing baseball against another Catholic school, and the coach decided not to start me, with no explanation. I was devastated and late in the game I took off my spikes, placed them under the bench, and slipped on my sneakers. In the last inning, the coach said I was pinch hitting for someone.

"No," I told him. "I'm done today."

Someone else pinch hit instead, the game ended, and the coach came up to me.

"Why didn't you pinch hit, Jamie?" he asked.

"I'm one of the best players on the team and you didn't let me play until the end of the game. I don't think that's very fair."

"I was just giving other boys a chance to play," replied the coach.

I rode my bike home and my dad met me on the first level of the house, inquiring how the game had gone. With frustration and anger, I recounted what had happened and he responded swiftly—with a short right jab to my face. I was stunned. A day or so later, he gave me a stern lecture on the ills of quitting and disrespecting my coach.

When Big Jim punched me, I was scared shitless, and there was no way I would hit him back. Combined with my fear of him, was my shame in disappointing him and my being upset that he wouldn't talk to me about my refusal to pinch hit. How could I live with this, if he wouldn't even hear my side of the story?

My father constantly stressed, "Work hard, do your best, be tough, be aggressive, kick ass and take names, be a man out there."

In my mind, following my dad's desire for me to be competitive had made me angry at my coach for not starting me. Then Dad had punched me in the face despite my following his directions. In disrespecting him in any fashion, one was asking for his wrath.

About this same time in grade school, several of my male friends and I were driven to a movie theater on a Saturday afternoon and watched cartoons and previews before the main attraction. In order to get a better view of the screen, we changed seats and made noise. The manager came to our location and severely reprimanded us for being rowdy.

"Boys," he said, loud enough for those around us to hear,

"if you can't act properly, you're going to have to leave."

"Sir," I replied, "we won't make any more noise. We're sorry."

"Young man," he said, "don't get mouthy with me."

"I'm not getting mouthy, sir. We just wanted to be able to see better."

"Don't talk back to me, buster. You and your friends are done—get out!"

"Sir, we haven't done anything wrong. We'll behave. We just want to watch the movie."

"You're done!" the manager barked, and led us out of the theater.

He called my father to come and pick us up, and 30 minutes later Big Jim arrived at the theater and interrogated us.

"Dad," I said, "we really didn't do anything wrong. We just moved seats before the movie started so we could see better. The manager became pissed off at us and threw us out."

"The manager," he said, "told me you were disrespectful and impolite to him and that's why you were told to leave."

"No way, Dad. I wasn't disrespectful at all to that man."

My buddies sat quietly in the back of the car, as my father dropped off each one in our neighborhood. When we arrived home, I was sent to my room. I felt I had been justified in defending myself and my friends with the manager, but again Dad didn't want to hear my side of the story, leaving me more confused and angry with his failure to believe his own son. I didn't say any of that to my dad. I went further inside myself, into my OCD and ritualistic compulsions, while trying to rid my brain of sexual obsessions. No one knew about this part of me, not even my closest friends. I had become superb at hiding my problems and my parents had become oblivious to my secret life.

There were instances when my mother and father displayed sincere love and pride in my accomplishments. When I was accepted into Georgetown Preparatory School to attend high school, Mom and Dad were thrilled. Together, they decided, much to their credit, to not accept a full tuition scholarship due to my academic grades and athletic abilities. Instead Jim and Bette requested Prep award the scholarship to a student more in need than our family. I was always very proud of my parents for this display of generosity and good will. In 2010, while being inducted into the Prep Hall of Fame, with my father present, I thanked Dad and my mother for the wonderful values they had taught me through their generous action.

I was a good kid in public, but in private, I was bombarded with anger and depression. In high school, I developed frequent head tics.

"Why are you shaking your head like that, Jamie?" my mother asked one day. "Do you realize you're doing that?"

"Yeah, Mom, I do."

What I would like to have said was: "I'm shaking my head so I don't kill myself. I have thoughts that won't go away. I'm going nuts and nobody seems to care."

I kept quiet and did my best to hide the tics.

In another situation, when in high school, on a late spring Saturday morning, I knocked on my parents' open bedroom door as they were lounging under the covers, reading and chatting.

"Mom and Dad," I said, "may I talk to you about something kind of important?"

"Sure, Jamie, come on in," Dad responded.

I sheepishly walked to the foot of my father's side of the king-sized bed, faced him, and said, "I have a concern that's been bothering me for a while. I need to see what you think."

"What is it, sweetheart?" my mother asked, as they set down their newspaper sections.

"I really enjoy and appreciate the car you gave me this year," I said. "It's great."

Big Jim had given me his 1964 black Ford Galaxie 500 convertible, with fire-engine red seats and a white top, a sweet set of wheels. He would repeat a similar scenario with all of his children.

"My car," I went on, looking at Dad, "is much nicer and newer than the cars a lot of the teachers at school are driving. I feel guilty about that. I am not sure I should be driving such a beautiful car as a sophomore in high school!"

"Jim," Dad said, "I've worked hard to provide your mother and you children with a nice home and a good life. There's nothing wrong with your driving a nice automobile. There's no shame in that."

"I know, Dad, but I feel guilty when teachers older than me, like Coach Fegan, don't have cars as nice as mine."

"Jamie," Mom said, "there's nothing to be ashamed of for having a good car. It gets you to school and you do errands in it for me and it's a big help when you pick up your brothers and sister. Remember that."

"You should never feel bad," my father added, "if you have

something someone else doesn't have, as long as you've worked hard to get it. You shouldn't worry about this, okay?"

Following a long, uncomfortable pause, I said, "Thanks, Mom and Dad for talking about this with me and thanks again for giving me the car."

Later, my mother told me that Big Jim was perplexed by my feeling I didn't deserve such a classy and expensive car. By now, my father and I were worlds apart and the car was just a symbol of that.

In speaking about the car with my parents, I was indirectly trying to explain to Dad about my virtues and values and my belief in practicing humility, empathy, sincerity and love. I did not believe in much of what I believed Dad most cherished: authority, power, wealth, social standing and success.

What I wanted to tell him was, "Dad, you and I are cut from the same cloth and some of our values are similar. We both regard highly: personal discipline, hard work, loyalty, dedication, mental and physical toughness, sportsmanship and competitiveness. But in many intimate, personal values, how we display our love, empathy, and compassion for others could not be more different. I have a mental illness which I fight against and strive to overcome every single day, but I refuse to allow it to make me less loving, less empathetic and less compassionate."

Then I would have said, "Dad, you have a mental illness and you don't care who gets hurt by it. You ignore this illness and storm ahead without caring how much you harm others in your way. To admit you're not perfect is to admit some kind of a problem or a level of defeat, and you're unwilling to do that."

What I was hoping for on that long ago Saturday morning was that my father would finally acknowledge to me, my mother and most importantly to himself, that he was not perfect or always right and not God. He was human and made mistakes like everyone else. He had an illness and if he had confronted it, he might have been able to control it.

What I most wanted to say was, "Dad, I love you with all my heart, but sometimes you're a real SOB to Mom, to me and many others, but you can change if you just try. Admit you have a problem and attack it with your inherent determination and perseverance. Mother comprehends that I have a problem, and has helped me. I just wish you could realize that I require your love and help to overcome my problem. Maybe you and I can help one another solve our problems. What do you think?"

But, of course, I said none of that.

On one hand I can count the number of times my father told me he loved me. The day he died, I was holding his hand as he breathed his last breath and I was still hoping he would change. He never took the time or made the effort to understand or discuss my OCD with me. He knew I was on medication and had been for years. He knew that I was seeing a psychiatrist and had been doing so for years, and knew that OCD was a mental illness. He never asked me about my OCD or my mental history. We never discussed my obsessions, compulsions, rituals or any aspect of the illness. As I grew older, he had no conception of what Betsy and I had experienced in over forty years of marriage, no clue. My mother occasionally inquired how I was feeling, but only in general terms. Over the decades, I talked with my youngest brother Robert about his and my OCD experiences, but not in much detail.

On the other hand, to my father's credit, he paid for many doctors who tried to assist me with my symptoms and paid tuition at multiple colleges for me to earn an education. He gave me possessions, but I wanted his love and affection. I might have benefited significantly from his sitting down and saying, "Jim, explain to me what OCD is and how it affects you? What can I do to help you beat this problem?"

There were ample opportunities to discuss topics of concern. Dad came alone to Colorado, even before my mother died in 2006, to attend high school and college graduations of our four children and when our second child was married in 2002. In 2012, about a year before his death, I traveled to New Jersey specifically to spend time with Dad. Earlier that year, I had gone home to honor his 90th birthday celebration at a formal dinner held in Atlantic City, where I made a short speech about his being a proud member of "America's Greatest Generation." My next trip east was just to check up on him and let him know I would be there for him when needed. That week together, he was uncharacteristically talkative and we enjoyed each other's company at several meals, with my sister Lisa accompanying us. For the first time ever, I took him to his doctor's appointments and we shopped for groceries. My final visit with him was a treat, but we never talked about OCD.

I began to lose faith in my dad when he never wanted to hear my side of the story when I encountered troubles. I think he lost faith in me as a productive, contributing adult in 1969, when I decided not to accept a congressional appointment to the U.S. Naval Academy—because my OCD symptoms were intensifying, frequently interrupting and controlling my life. From that time until I was sixty-five, my life deteriorated, including my personal life, professional career and long-term goals and aspirations, so often foiled because of OCD.

It is only because of my wife that I am still here today, fighting the good fight, rather than residing in a mental institution.

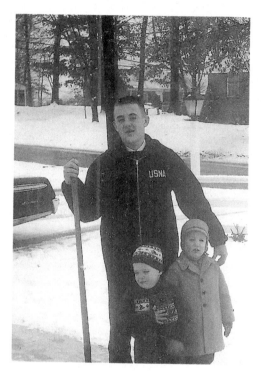

Author and two youngest brothers
Kensington, MD, mid 60's

# Chapter IV

# Running Away

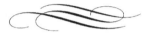

*A*t fourteen, I began attending an all-male, exclusive, parochial preparatory high school, Georgetown Prep, founded in 1789. This was my choice to attend Prep, as a peer idol of mine from grade school had gone to this school a few years earlier. Tuition per year was $800, a significant sum for a government-employed professional with seven children, but Big Jim and Mom were happy to pay the tuition and fees, and they were very proud of me.

I was ecstatic, believing I would continue earning good grades, compete in numerous sports, and develop many lasting friendships. From there, I would be accepted into the U.S. Naval Academy. During my first semester, I adapted well to the three hours of homework every night, struggling somewhat with algebra and Latin, but making the academic honor roll the first two grading quarters. I met many wonderful friends, made a name for myself playing football, and attended one or two school dances with a date, but girls were not that important to me, because I had not met the right girl for me.

By late November and early December, I was losing

my edge in academics. Concentration became far more difficult and I experienced regular migraine headaches, usually when attempting to study. I was afraid of failing, losing confidence and sliding into depression. At home over Christmas vacation, I felt trepidation about returning to my classes. When it was time to go back to school, I had already decided against this.

That Sunday evening, I departed our house about 11:00 p.m. and walked to a grade school friend's tree fort in thickly wooded Rock Creek Park, a mile from my parent's address. This gave me shelter for the longest and coldest night of my life. Nearly frozen, I returned home around 8:30 a.m. on Monday morning, after a night of deep reflection and very little sleep. I had a thick hardback book with me, the pages I burned to stay warm, but I was still terribly cold.

"What was wrong with me," I asked myself over and over as I sat in the tree fort and searched for answers. "What have I done to deserve this misery?"

Rather than using language, I ran away for a night, at the end of Christmas break, to show my parents that I was experiencing headaches, depression and anxiety, which was impeding my academic performance.

Afraid to talk to them, I had bolted.

When I made it home, my parents were relieved but in shock. My father made arrangements for the three of us to see a family friend, a well-known and well-respected local pediatrician, and we visited him the next day. This began my life-long odyssey of consulting a plethora of pediatricians and later psychiatrists who, in multiple cases, were sincere and caring, but had absolutely no idea what was troubling me. I was a human time bomb, waiting for the right trigger to explode. Would I lash out at fellow students and hurt them—or one of my younger siblings? Or would I punch myself in the face until it looked as if I'd lost a fist fight? I did this more than once in college.

My life as an adolescent and young adult was hellish during what should have been some of the most rewarding and joyous days of my life. OCD eviscerates and destroys one's sense of well-being. Hitting oneself repeatedly in the face is not normal. Yet when I could not dismiss repetitive obsessions from my mind, I reverted to such behavior. Or I punched holes in a wall with my fists, threw furniture or took a kitchen knife and pressed it against my neck, threatening to cut myself.

"I did not commit a sin; I did not commit a sin," I whispered over and over and over during these episodes, while slapping myself in the face to make thoughts of sin go away. If they persisted, I might go out to the garage or down in the recreation room and throw tools or glasses or books or whatever was at hand. I kicked my own car and dented it, hurled pictures or mirrors, bats and baseballs, lawn furniture–anything to make the obsessions and compulsions disappear, but that did not happen.

Two or three times, I destroyed personal property at home construction sites as a youth. Once, my friends and I threw stones and broke numerous windows in a new home. At another house, we knocked down a newly-built cinder block wall, causing a hundred dollars of damage. I once talked my younger brother and our cousin into going out into the bay which held a wild-bird preserve. In a mad dash, we smashed dozens and dozens of baby bird eggs in this sanctuary. As I write this, I can actually feel the relief of pressure within my body and the pleasure I experienced by exerting my power to destroy these objects. I felt no pain, no guilt at the time I did this. I was glad to be able to do something to feel this relief, even though it was terribly wrong behavior. Freedom came with exercising my choice to do wrong.

I was acting out like this because in the rest of my life I had to be perfect for my dad and my religion—a perfect gentleman, as my father's son and a Catholic school child, and I was sick of this structure. I wanted to kick my father's butt, yet that would have been committing a mortal sin, so better for walls and windows and birds to suffer.

Having a pall—or an impulse toward violence—descend upon you at any time or place was debilitating and unnerving. Not knowing when this would occur made my life almost not worth living. One escape was sleeping and I did so excessively at college and at home as well; weekends were just for sleeping. Later, I slept all the time when our young children took naps, and I am now saddened by how many thousands of hours I squandered due to the effects of OCD.

Following the initial consultation with the pediatrician, I continued to see him regularly, once a week, for a month or so. The doctor talked about my "scrupulosity problem" being one cause of my symptoms. My headaches and inability to concentrate on my studies, he said, were driven by being overly meticulous about sinning or not sinning.

My parents spoke with my school Headmaster and the Dean of Students. Both were understanding and supportive, and I was permitted to return to school, but I didn't fare well the remainder of my freshman year. Each time I sat down to study, the headaches were back. I tried taking breaks, studying in different locations and with other classmates, but I earned D's and F's in every course for the remainder of my freshman year.

I thought I was having a nervous breakdown, but much later in life I would learn that the stress of beginning in a new school, with three hours of homework every evening, brought on migraine headaches due to a hormonal, physiological response to the stress. I was fourteen and in the middle of puberty. Within six months, the migraines would disappear and never return.

The summer following my freshman year, my family rented a home in Ocean City, N.J., as one set of my grandparents owned a cottage located right on the water. Through sheer good fortune or divine intervention, I met and befriended the girl next door to my grandparents, Betsy, my wife of almost half a century. What are the chances that the first woman you ever kissed becomes the love of your life? My headaches disappeared, which made sense because I was not involved with school or homework. I went water skiing and enjoyed the summer with my favorite cousin, John, and my good friend, Billy, along with my future wife and her girlfriends. Life was good again. Whenever I have kept busy and been productively occupied, my OCD incidents have subsided to some degree.

From Betsy:

*It was the summer of 1964 and my parents had just purchased a house at the Jersey shore. One of our first days there, my dad and I were looking out the kitchen window when this young boy walked alongside the house next door. I turned to my father and said, "Do you see that guy? I'm going to marry him one day!" My dad didn't say much, but I meant what I'd said. It would never have occurred to me what an important role my father would play in my eventual marriage.*

*I had a great relationship with my father—a warm, kind, compassionate, and easy-to-be-with person. A self-made man, he'd quit school at fourteen, lied about his age, and went to work at the Tastykake Baking Company in Philadelphia, Pa., sweeping floors to support his mother and sister (his father had passed away when he was seven). He continued working there for the next 35 years and became the vice-president. Admired and widely respected, he knew almost every employee by his or her first name. Shortly after the president of the company died, my father was in line for this position, but it was a family-owned business and they decided to bring in a relative to run the company, who knew absolutely nothing about baking. He clashed with my dad, who was in a bind because when becoming the VP, he had signed a contract that he couldn't work for another baking company. Things began to deteriorate at work and he turned to alcohol, basically drinking himself to death over the next ten years.*

*During that decade, my sister and brother moved on, with the former at nursing school and the latter in military service. That left my mother and me, and things were not good at home. My mother went away for six weeks to take care of her sister in Arizona and when she returned she took a job with the IRS doing tax returns, working the three-to-eleven p.m. shift and leaving me alone with my father and his drinking. I never spoke of any of this to my friends and they never suspected that anything was amiss in our household. In those last years with my dad, I developed a self-defense mechanism that allowed me to ignore or forget what was happening around me and that strategy has stayed with me ever since. I used this strategy to protect myself so I too led a kind of "secret life," like Jim.*

*I never thought that I'd thank my dad for being an alcoholic, but because of this mechanism I was able to cope with Jim's OCD much more so than the average individual. He had all the characteristics of my dad, but without the alcohol. He was warm, compassionate, kind, and easy to be with and talk to. That first summer we instantly connected because he wasn't like a lot of the boys I went to high school with, but much more. He taught me how to water ski, which we did every day, and he'd come to the boardwalk and accompany me home from my job each night. We talked for hours and he became my best friend. At that time, I don't remember him having any OCD problems, but he was just fun to be around.*

*We dated for eight years before getting married. Even though I came to realize that he had issues, I knew that I wanted to be with him forever. I saw what my mother had gone through with my dad and didn't think anything could be worse than that, so I felt certain that I could handle whatever was coming with Jim. I could see through his problems to the person he really was—just as I did with my father. The difference was that Jim truly tried to get better, which my father never did once the drinking began. He just became worse.*

*With Jim, I felt there could be a solution—a light at the end of the tunnel—if we could only find it, and we eventually did. That never happened with my father; he basically gave up and I couldn't forgive him for that.*

On August 1, 1964, I said good-bye to Betsy and returned to school for football camp and the opportunity to make the varsity team as a sophomore, a very difficult goal. My headaches had gone, and I was anxious to prove myself mentally and physically in football, which allowed me to take out my anxiety and frustration through contact on the field, something I reveled in.

Through three weeks of football boot camp, and through hard work, perseverance and determination, I not only made the varsity team, but earned a starting position. I overcame open, quarter-size blisters on both heels to compete on a squad that went undefeated and became league champions.

Sophomore year I carried on a serious relationship by phone with Betsy. Until now I had been deathly afraid of calling girls. My grades improved slightly: F's in Latin, but D's and C's in most other classes, earning my one and only A in high school in biology. I took the driving test, passed with perfect scores, and was given my own car for travelling to school. I was also feeling good about my faith and hadn't experienced any problems while attending confession. The expanding Vietnam War, the draft, student demonstrations and the Civil Rights movement swirled around me, but I remained relatively content for the last three years of high school.

My junior year I began visibly nodding my head to one side or the other—to make myself stop obsessing on an OCD thought. I tried to hide this tic and my parents and siblings noticed yet never said too much about it. The number of times I subconsciously shook my head varied, with possibly five to fifteen incidents per day, and this lasted at least six months. After I made a conscious effort to stop this, it eventually worked.

I also began brushing my hair over and over, then messing up my hair and re-brushing it. This was a daily ritual and might consume several minutes or more each time it occurred. My hand-washing ritual started in high school and has remained with me ever since.

Before going out to football practice each day, I would put on my cleats and I would silently recite the following prayer: "Jesus, please give me the strength, courage, determination, confidence, and pride to do my best today. Please protect everyone from serious injury. Amen."

I had to say this perfectly or make myself repeat it. If I had to repeat the prayer more than twice, I might find myself murmuring it out loud, especially if I had not said it perfectly the first time. I also developed a streak of self-righteousness. Beginning in eighth grade, if a peer or teammate did something I considered immoral or wrong, I would retaliate verbally or physically. During a school ceremony at our church, a schoolmate gave the finger to another student. After leaving church, I reprimanded my friend, saying this behavior was sinful. He balked, so I punched him, feeling that was my responsibility.

Riding the bus to school one day as a sophomore, I saw a freshman from my parochial grade school being bullied by his classmate. I whispered to the bus driver James that I would take care of the problem, and I walked calmly back to where the bully was taunting the young man verbally and physically pointing his finger into the chest of the student. Forty-six years later at an athletic awards ceremony at our high school, the bullied student came up to me. I recognized him, but had forgotten his name. He introduced himself as Dr. So and So and introduced his wife, also a physician.

He smiled and said, "Do you remember that day on the bus, when Bully X was bothering me? You came down the aisle, could not speak, and grabbed him by the shirt and the knot of his tie. You lifted him out of the seat and he turned white and didn't say a word. You told him that if he ever bothered me again, you'd kick the living shit out of him. Then you asked him if he understood and he shook his head yes. You dropped him and you both went back to your seats. He never bothered me again. My mother called the Dean of Discipline at school to voice her concern. The dean told my mother that she didn't have to worry anymore: "Jimmy Juliana had addressed the situation and there would no longer be any bullying."

The doctor looked me right in the eye, with emotion in his eyes, and said he had always wanted to share this story with me. I thanked him and expressed how wonderful it was seeing him and meeting his wife. We chatted a few more moments before going our separate ways. His sentiments meant much more to me than the award I received later in the evening, during my induction into the Georgetown Preparatory School Athletic Hall of Fame.

Athletics have always been an integral part of my life and especially in my dealings with OCD. Prior to meeting Betsy and her influence becoming so important to me, I found participating in sports to be literally a Godsend. Had I not enjoyed and thrived in participation in athletics, I might not have survived adolescence and my early years with OCD. Sports gave me both a physical and emotional outlet for my anxiety, fear and frustration. I especially appreciated and enjoyed football; the physical contact provided a release and relief for my ever-present anger due to my OCD obsessions and compulsions.

When I began high school, the sports camaraderie and my striving for excellence as an athlete provided me with a sense of stability and strength. Because I was failing miserably as a student, athletics became even more important. To offset a devastating freshman year academically, I compensated with athletic achievements and made many solid friendships. Despite my "secret life" of depression and deep anxiety, I earned respect for my prowess as a competitor and for striving to be a kind and sincere person.

As a senior in high school, I had made it through three years of non-stop encounters with OCD symptoms, while barely managing to keep my head above water in the classroom. I had also developed a very real and meaningful relationship with Betsy, but then something happened at school that challenged my sense of self and my stability. During our senior football season, I heard from a boarding student friend that a Jesuit scholastic, a priest/teacher in training, had said this to some other boarding students whom he proctored and mentored as a live-in resident: "That Juliana is an animal. They should keep him in a cage during the week and only let him out on game days to play."

Learning that these words had been uttered by a faculty member, I was devastated emotionally. What would my younger brother, Patrick, a freshman, think of this? What about my teammates and peers—or my parents? Fifty-three years later, I cannot fathom why this teacher would have made such a public statement in front of other students about someone he did not really know and had never had in class? My conscience, already terribly convoluted from obsessions and compulsions related to guilt, mortal sins and the evils of all sex, was overwhelmed with thoughts of being worthless, stupid and beyond salvation.

How could this have happened? I was co-captain of the varsity football team and well-liked by my peers and especially by the senior class members. I was trying my best in school and was a member of the Student Conduct Committee at school. I was doing everything I could to be a good Catholic and a good human being, but evidently a small group of Jesuit novitiates believed I was unworthy of being a Prep student-athlete.

Until recently, I never really considered what my parents must have thought when I related this news to them. At the time, my parents, both devout Catholics, were in disbelief that a Jesuit novitiate, a priest in training, would utter such words about their son. I remember my father asking me what I wanted him to do regarding the situation. I said he did not have to do anything. I was going to go to school the next day and kick the shit out of this teacher. In a rare moment of paternal love and compassion for me, Dad said, "Jim, please do not go back to school and confront this guy. You will get expelled from school. You have worked too hard to graduate. You should graduate. For your mother's sake and mine don't do anything to him."

I complied with my father's wishes, because I respected and loved him and always wanted to please him. Yet not confronting the man physically and kicking his ass seemed rather unmanly on my part. But Dad was right and many years ago, I forgave the young Jesuit.

At graduation eight months later, I was awarded the Alumni Memorial Medal in commemoration of deceased alumni: "…awarded in recognition of sportsmanship, manliness, competitive spirit and the other virtues of the Christian gentleman as displayed in the field of athletic endeavor during the Junior and Senior Years." That medal and its inscription hang in my den today. I cherish this award as much as I do my high school diploma.

Thank you, Dad, for being wiser than your oldest son.

I am proud of my parents for how they handled this unfortunate situation and proud of myself overcoming this adversity in my young life. Back then, I was simply trying to survive my "secret life" with my undiagnosed OCD, by putting all of my passion and energy into athletics. I had made it through this particular situation, but there was always another challenge ahead.

As a collage freshman one evening, I was walking home across campus at the University of New Hampshire, after attending a movie with my two roommates, (I was 5'8" and weighed 178 pounds). My 6'5", 265-pound offensive lineman roommate pulled out his penis and urinated on the grass, with no regard for passing students, some of the students were female.

"Hey, asshole," I said, "there are women walking by here. Have some manners."

The offensive lineman sucker punched me, and I fell to the ground, but kept quiet as we continued walking to our dorm. My roommates walked into our room, but I lingered outside. Directly across the hallway was a coke machine, and I grabbed an empty, seven-ounce, green Coke bottle and broke off the bottom in an adjoining sink. I rushed across the hall into our room, where my large roommate sat on the bottom bunk bed. Gripping his hair with my left hand, I shoved back his head and placed the broken edge of the bottle up to his neck.

"You ever touch me again," I screamed, "I'll kill you!"

I held the sharp edges of the glass bottle at his neck for at least 30 seconds, making sure he understood the message. I do not remember if I drew blood, but the two campus policemen who responded a short while later did not pursue me, as I had walked outside to cool off. My lineman roommate never messed with me again. No one in the dorm did.

The campus newspaper, after my having carried out several campus pranks with several other students, nicknamed this anonymous prankster student, "Mad Dog," and the editor of the paper called the group of guys I led, "Mad Dog's Marauders," a diversion from my OCD.

And a time bomb waiting to be triggered.

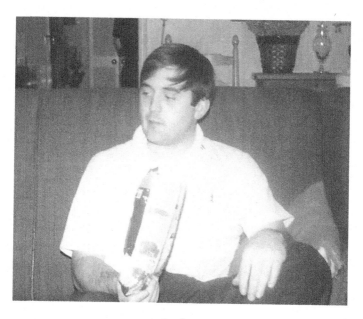

Author
Rockville, MD, early 70's

# Chapter V

# The War Inside

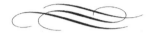

$B$etsy graduated from high school and moved to Washington, D.C. to attend college at the beginning of my junior year in high school. Despite her witnessing some of my worse OCD incidents and knowing how irrational my behavior could become, we became romantically involved. The hair brushing, hand washing, head tics, not walking on lines on the sidewalk and perfect praying before football practice all intensified. My behavior, not yet diagnosed as OCD, worsened considerably during late adolescence, Betsy became the most important person and confidant in my life. She quickly supplanted my mother, now on her way to becoming an alcoholic.

From Betsy:

*I lived in Philadelphia and Jamie lived in Washington, D. C. After I graduated from high school, I went to a school in Washington to become a medical secretary. Jamie and I soon continued our friendship/courtship. He, from the beginning, was such a warm, polite, caring and good-looking guy that I think I immediately fell in love with him. I went to all of his football games. We dated during his junior and senior years, went to dances, parties and I got to know most of his friends. We actually double-dated often with another football player and his girlfriend, and they later married after us. I began a job at The National Institutes of Health in Bethesda, Md. and lived in an apartment with a couple of friends, and Jim and I continued to date.*

*After graduating from high school, Jim attended Bullis Prep for one year to prepare for entrance into the Naval Academy. Then he decided to go to The University of New Hampshire. At that time I moved back to Philadelphia, in a way to be closer to him. I worked at Temple Hospital for three years before we eventually became engaged.*

*I always knew Jim had a "problem." God knows his mother certainly tried to break us up, because she didn't think I could handle it. Or at least that was my point of view. My father was the Vice President of TastyKake, a baking company, in Philadelphia. He had some horrific issues at work and because of that, had a nervous breakdown and became an alcoholic. I think watching my mother and how she stood by my dad and took care of him let me see that if I wanted to, I too could help Jamie in any way I could. I can't say it was easy. There were lots of times that I wasn't sure I could handle what I had taken on. But I knew down deep inside that Jim was an amazing person, a good guy and could be a great father, husband, friend and teacher and somehow had been dealt a really bad hand. I just kept hoping that one day things would get better for him.*

For eleven years of my education, the nuns in my grade school, the Sisters of Charity, and the Jesuits in high school taught the Catholic faith and its doctrines to me and millions of other young Catholics, using the Baltimore Catechism. Students learned the meaning of the Ten Commandments, the significance of the seven sacraments, and the specific way in which a Catholic could acquire additional spiritual assistance and help—through Baptism, receiving the Holy Eucharist and Penance, through admitting one's sins and receiving absolution in confession. Nuns and priests placed great emphasis on our making mistakes, sinning and being forgiven for these sins by God through going to confession. Many of my Catholic friends and acquaintances have also experienced, in adulthood, a personal overemphasis and problems with sin and confession as I have.

A person's sexuality forms during childhood and with the onset of puberty, and this maturation often collides with one's religious mores, especially if you are raised within Catholicism's ardent rules and regulations. For strict Catholic children, the complex process is multiplied several times. Now add a phobia, later defined as a chemical imbalance in one's brain, and one can face a debilitating set of circumstances, beyond the control of a child or young adolescent. That was my circumstance.

Totally overwhelmed emotionally and psychologically best describes my state of mind when dealing with unwanted thoughts, obsessions, ritualistic actions and compulsions. An unrelenting and oppressive fear and despair came over me when talking with my mother and trying to sort out why I was thinking what I was thinking or convincing myself that I was not committing mortal sins. Because my Catholic faith was so important in my life and my family's life, and because my religion teachers had instilled sacred principles of right and wrong in my brain, how could this young child react inappropriately to looking at a picture of a naked woman?

While my obsessions grew, I spent a significant amount of time trying to maintain a close, personal relationship with Jesus and my faith. I continued serving mass at our school chapel and served in high school on the Student Conduct Committee. My focus was on athletics, Betsy and a handful of close, supportive friends. I was the only student in my Latin class senior year excused from studying the ancient language. My German grades were charity D's. As a junior, I failed chemistry, and was consistently in the bottom 10% of my class. I had to attend an extra year of college prep school to raise my SAT scores and GPA to qualify for the Naval Academy.

I also experienced some successes; I was the president of my junior class at Prep and President of the Student Council at Bullis Prep School. I was co-captain of the football team at both schools and received numerous athletic honors and trophies, but OCD was always with me. Our football team at Bullis Prep competed against college freshman teams, some of them excellent. Midway into the season, I developed a horrible sensation on the field, which felt as if pins were being poked into my eyeballs. It happened in practice and games. I'd rub my eyes and blink, but nothing helped. It was highly distracting and clearly affected my performance. The sensation finally stopped, but over the years has reoccurred for short durations. I have no idea why this happened. Another phobia possibly?

I earned my diploma from Georgetown Prep, finishing 57th academically out of 60 students. And I was turned down by all dozen colleges to which I applied. After the year at Bullis, I was accepted into the Naval Academy, but declined to accept my appointment, in part, because of my OCD and because I had not passed college chemistry and calculus while at Bullis. The University of Massachusetts accepted me for their summer semester—after a business associate of my father intervened. I attended classes for two weeks, then suddenly quit, returning home and working that summer for a trucking company, unloading and loading freight into fifty-foot-long containers in brutally hot weather in Virginia.

OCD has always affected my employment history, just as it had everything else in which I was involved. I would labor diligently all summer, but when it was time to return to school, I would quit my job, and tell no one what I was doing. No notice to my bosses or co-workers—nothing. I found this technique much less stressful than speaking face-to-face with a supervisor. My inability to discuss important issues with authority figures was constant, in adolescence and into middle age, when leaving teaching positions and beyond.

A couple of times as a young man, I made plans to take a vacation trip with a friend and never showed up for the engagement or called the person, because I despised using phones and still do today. Sometimes, I felt like a mute person, almost incapable of explaining myself or my unusual actions.

Behind everything was my secret, ongoing war with OCD. The following ritual is one I have performed every time I have showered for the past fifteen years or more. It may strike you as crazy unless you are an OCD sufferer or a physician treating OCD patients. In the shower I must wash myself in a very strict, uniform order and procedure. If the order deviates at all, I must begin washing myself over again. The ritual consumes my entire shower, as well as the time it takes to dry off, which is a continuation of the compulsion and requires a specific ritual of its own. This compulsion can last much longer than it normally takes to dry off after a shower. I have finally broken this compulsion recently, since I began seeing Dr. James Gallagher.

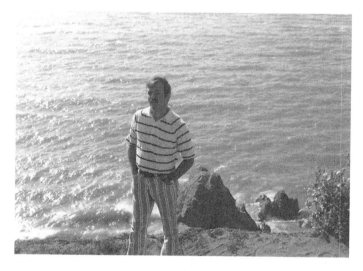

Author
San Francisco, CA, 1971

# Chapter VI

# Early Adulthood and College

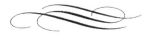

$A$t nineteen, I left D.C. to attend the University of New Hampshire. I wanted one more opportunity to play college football and thought moving away from home might help me overcome my still undiagnosed OCD. Creating some unfamiliarity in my life might possibly be useful.

I walked-on in football, which means I made the freshman team without a scholarship. I took four, three-hour classes, the minimum to remain eligible to compete in athletics. My OCD incidents kept coming often and were again related to feeling that I was committing mortal sins and hurting God. That fall while scrimmaging, I grabbed the face mask of a varsity player, because he was hitting me after the whistle had blown. This escalated into nasty language and a few punches. I was kicked out of the drill, took off my helmet, and threw it at a varsity coach. Fortunately, the helmet didn't hit the coach, and I was allowed to remain on the team.

I rarely studied, even during mandatory study hall for the athletes, and had no focus, no motivation and no reason to concentrate on my classes. I was depressed much of the time and deeply missed Betsy. She visited twice during the semester, but that left me more depressed once she was gone. I saw her over Christmas break and my head tics returned. My OCD was like a living virus or entity within me, flaring up when I was unhappy, almost unbearable at times. On occasion, I was convinced that I was literally possessed by the devil. Anyone with my sexual thoughts or level of frustration and anger must be possessed, I thought often. A supernatural force had to be inside of me to make me think and act the way I did.

In thousands of instances, I could be enjoying a beautiful day and with no warning at all, a sexual thought would invade my mind. Hell would break loose within me, as I tried to eliminate this thought of sex. Once I succeeded in pushing the unwanted thought aside, my obsessive thought became: did I commit a mortal sin by thinking about having sex with some woman? Am I going to hell? Must I seek absolution? Am I a pervert for having had this thought?

I would begin to perspire and my temperature rose, along with my heartbeat. I grew tense, embarrassed and frustrated. Sometimes I had not heard anything anyone had said for the past 10, 15 or maybe 30 minutes in class while the professor lectured. I would attempt to maintain my calm when I had just thought of some random immoral act in which I would normally never conceive. I had just spent half an hour trying to convince myself that I had not committed a mortal sin, leaving me mentally and emotionally drained, ready to lose my temper.

I am Italian and we are emotional people who talk and gesture with our hands and bodies. We are passionate about our family, our faith, politics and often sports. Italian, non-Italian, any normal man or woman is going to become angry or disturbed if his/her daily routine is suddenly and inexplicably turned upside down by a random thought or behavior, which completely overwhelms that person's mind and actions.

From adolescence on, I had thoughts of suicide. Many times I imagined speeding in my car and driving off the road into a tree or bridge. As a young man, I often held a knife or fork up to my neck and pictured myself pushing the utensil into my throat. Then in a perverse way, I would think, "I cannot commit suicide. Suicide is a mortal sin, and if I commit a mortal sin, my soul goes straight to hell!" On at least two occasions, I became so angry that I pulled the steering wheel in my car so violently I broke it. Fortunately, the car was in park at the time.

At New Hampshire University, I once led "Mad Dog's Marauders" in taking dormitory lounge furniture out onto the grassy square in front of several dormitory buildings, and stacking wooden chairs, tables and any other combustible materials into a large pile. I had acquired an over-sized can of lighter fluid, which I squirted all over the furniture, newspapers and any other flammable items which were piled together. The ensuing huge bon fire, along with hundreds of crazed students throwing their clothes into the conflagration, then running and jumping over sections of the blaze, made for an excellent story in the campus daily. Once again, I somehow managed to escape retribution by the campus police department. This was probably the most enjoyable and memorable event of my six months on campus—thumbing my nose both at authority and my ever-present OCD.

That was my state of mind for one semester in 1968. At that point, the U.S. Selective Service System instituted the lottery to do away with inequities of the draft for the Vietnam War. I remember watching television in my college dormitory lounge as ping pong balls with the 366 days of the year painted on them were picked out of a round cage. The lottery official read the number of the date out loud and each birth date represented who would be drafted first, second and so on. My birthday was the thirteenth one chosen, and I suddenly realized that evening that I would eventually be drafted. I quit college and returned home to D. C. in late February 1969; my GPA after one semester 1.0: two C's, a D and an F. I had lettered in freshman football, but my football career was over.

Coming home was one of the most depressing experiences of my life; I was a failure with few options. My parents were disappointed and had no idea how to help me. I found a full-time job at Bethesda Naval Hospital, had other part-time work, and was making sufficient money not to rely on my folks, except for a bedroom. I was out of the house and away from the family as much as possible. Again, Betsy was the most positive and stabilizing part of my life. She lived three hours away in Philly, so we took turns commuting to visit one another. Had I not had her as a friend and confidant, I may well have committed suicide, despite my belief that it would be a ticket to hell.

The head tics had returned and I experienced constant OCD incidents throughout each day. My peer group did a lot of drinking and a few of them were heavily into drugs.

The Vietnam War, peace demonstrations, anti-war protests and race riots took place often in D.C. And yet, with all of the constant commotion, I maintained a semblance of sanity and equilibrium. My full-time work on the grounds of the VA hospital allowed me to witness the ravages of war, by interacting with horribly wounded and injured veterans. I thanked God for keeping me from these horrors. My closest co-worker was a young black man, a few years older than me, an ex-convict, trying to start a better life. We talked about race relations, the war and many life-topics.

I learned much from this young man, starting with the depth of the hurt he felt from prejudice, hearing nasty prison stories of sexual abuse and strained race relations. He talked about his upbringing in poverty and his fear of returning to prison, which drove him to work hard and make more productive use of his talents. He was honest and open and explained to me how some of my own ideas were negative and racist. I learned a lot about myself and my own misconceptions of blacks in the six months we shared.

With him, as with everyone else, I worked very diligently to hide my OCD. Longtime friends and acquaintances have often told me after I have shared a part of my secret life with them: "I never knew you had a problem with that." In my college classes or when working, I spent so much time and energy disguising my symptoms that I was usually exhausted at night from my prolonged, heated arguments within my mind or because of my efforts to dismiss an OCD thought. If I noticed an attractive coed walking into a lecture hall, I might walk by her, smile, say hello, and flirt a little, maybe complementing her on her tan.

Then I might begin to obsess about her and had difficulty stopping this. I had allowed myself a moment of pleasure and was now accusing myself of committing a mortal sin. My conscience said "mortal sin;" my brain said "no big deal, get on with class." This fight inside me could last the remainder of the hour-long class, leaving me angry and spent.

I have experienced thousands and thousands of similar incidents, where I took 20 minutes or more to rectify or settle an inner conflict within my mind, so I could go on with my daily routine. The hours I have wasted are incalculable and the time lost has to be close to years. Add to that all the time I have spent oversleeping trying to avoid OCD incidents. Plus the depression and resulting medications for treatment—which often brought on drowsiness—I have slept through entire days, except to go to the bathroom.

While working at the VA hospital, I was accepted into a local junior college in Maryland, where I earned A's and B's, including another perfect A in biology. I felt comfortable at the school and even though the OCD was present, the incidents were not as frequent or severe. My relationship with Betsy had strengthened considerably, and for the first time I could be myself around a person of the opposite sex without feeling awkward or ill at ease. We talked for hours about our goals and aspirations, and I shared some of my OCD experiences with her.

In early 1970, I received the long-expected invitation from my draft board to appear for a physical. I recall walking around in my underwear, dark socks and shoes with hundreds of other scared shitless teenagers and young men, many of them more freaked out than I was. Scores of guys meandered through a large warehouse, pushed and prodded by male nurses and directed along to all types of doctors and technicians. This lasted for much of the day, as every inch of our bodies was examined and reviewed. The climax came when I was instructed to speak with a psychiatrist, the one doctor I had eagerly anticipated seeing. He was honest and sincere and appeared much more interested in me as a person than anyone else had all day.

I had been carrying around, stuck into my shorts, a copy of a letter from one of my closest friend's father, who was a pediatrician. He knew my history of headaches and studying problems in high school and my personal difficulties at college, including the fits of anger and frustration and physical confrontations. The letter read, "I believe Mr. Juliana is unfit for military service, due to severe psychological problems, related to depression and anger..." His words saved me from being drafted into the military and possibly being killed or maimed in Vietnam. A few months prior to my physical, I had ventured into a U.S. Marine recruiting station to enlist. A close friend from grade school, a U.S. Army Green Beret, had accompanied me and talked me out of this at the last moment. Then the doctor's letter saved me once again. From this time forward, my military draft status was 4F, unfit for military service, a badge I have worn with both shame and relief.

While I attended junior college, a family friend secured for me an excellent paying position with the federal government at the U. S. Capitol. My closest co-workers were three former Vietnam vets, who'd retained their health and their limbs, along with considerable cynicism and criticism for their government. Two were married with children and all were eight or ten years older than me and had experienced combat and other scenarios which I knew little or nothing about. They teased me incessantly for my blind patriotism and idealism, but were never mean or unforgiving. I was comfortable around them and in their company. My OCD rarely bothered me then. Their questioning of the status quo and disdain for many rules and regulations eased my symptoms; I was happier and more carefree than in years.

These veterans were understandably angry with their government for having put them into life and death situations. Many of their concerns were legitimate, even to a conservative like me, and we argued and disagreed during lengthy discussions, yet remained friends. They treated me as an equal, despite my not being a vet or anti-war and honored my values and ideas. They were not authoritative toward me, which seemed to lead to my OCD not bothering me as much. My obsessions and compulsions were far fewer working with these vets, and my secret life was temporarily put on hold.

In recent years, I've made a new friend through my volunteer work with veterans. This man, whom I will call John, served several tours of duty in Vietnam in the First Calvary of the US Army, and for the past 45 years has suffered significantly from Post-Traumatic Stress Disorder. He's been in and out of VA hospitals and prescribed multiple medications. Like me, he has had difficulty keeping jobs and experienced brushes with the law. John has a secret life perpetrated by PTSD, just as I have mine with OCD. I realize that his war experiences, as well as his feelings and emotions from them, may be much more serious and complex than my obsessions and compulsions. Yet being around him, I can empathize with his frustration and anxiety, his pain and suffering. While OCD is not PTSD, I suspect both share many of the same after-effects, including deep depression, anxiety and guilt. Because of my OCD, I have more compassion for people like John than I otherwise would have.

Looking back, I believe that my OCD was not the critical factor in my problems with authority, but rather it was the stress, frustration and depression that came from trying to cope with those in charge. Likewise, my Catholicism has never been the primary stimulus for my symptoms. Individuals can be scrupulous about their religious beliefs without having OCD, but the chemical imbalance in my brain did not make that possible for me.

After three semesters of junior college, I applied to George Washington University where I was accepted. I felt proud of myself and confident in my academic abilities. I scheduled a full-load of fifteen hours of classes and began coaching freshman football at my high school—my passion for the next forty years. The head freshman coach, Bobby, a Prep grad, owned a restaurant and bar, where I went to work as a waiter and bartender. Once again, when I was busy and productive like this, the OCD incidents were kept to a minimum.

Betsy and I continued to date and my grades remained better than average, except for speech class, which I hated and in which I earned an F. I tried out for the varsity baseball team at GW and made the squad as a seldom-used, utility player, but the camaraderie and physical exertion were good for me. The longer I coached into the future, the more comfortable I became at public speaking and giving motivational talks. Standing in front of students for the 28 years I taught, and presenting facts and information was never easy for me, but I forced myself to appear relaxed.

By the summer of 1971, after three more college semesters, I was faced with the most serious decision of my life: Was I going to marry Betsy? She agreed to my plan: I took a job in the state of Washington, working for the federal government, the National Park Service. Exploring the country with my brother Pat and my brother's best friend Willie, both college athletes, I would have the summer to decide if I was ready for marriage—given everything I knew about myself—and if so, I would return to school and our wedding in 1972. I headed west for a life-changing adventure.

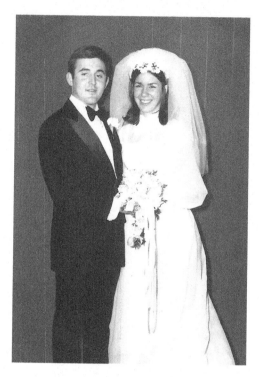

Betsy and Jim
Immaculate Conception Catholic Church
Jenkintown, PA; January 8, 1972

# Chapter VII

# Marriage

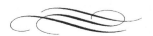

*A*s I left for the Olympic National Park in Washington, my OCD was as strong as ever. If I saw a naked woman in a movie, my conscience told me I had committed a mortal sin by looking at the woman, and I would have to look away. I would start a back and forth argument between my conscience and my brain, as my heart rate rose and I began to perspire. Just when my brain might have convinced my conscience I hadn't sinned, my conscience would say that I had wanted to commit a mortal sin. This compulsion might take 30 minutes or longer to resolve the question in my mind, but almost always my conscience won out over my brain. In the end, I was a sinner.

These inner arguments left me so angry and violent that I threw objects—a phone, a vase, a framed picture or a glass. I punched walls with my fists or head. If someone was with me, like Betsy or my mother or a friend, they would often think I was angry at them, but I was enraged at my OCD, like an evil power within me with complete control over my thoughts. The older I became the angrier and more frustrated I was at being incapable of dismissing what came into my mind. If I could have isolated the evil entity, I would have beaten it to death with my fists.

That was my state of mind when I left for the west coast in May of 1971. Living away from my parents, their authority and any emphasis on money, prestige and influence, I could perhaps gain control of the OCD incidents. I hoped experiencing an adventure in other parts of the country with people I enjoyed might be the remedy. I loved my brother Pat and this adventure became the trip of a lifetime, but I could not run away from OCD. The challenge was to control and manage it.

Driving across the flat plains of South Dakota, I witnessed the largest and most magnificent and colorful rainbow I have ever seen, stretching across the entire sky. We camped under more stars than I had imagined existed and one day we drove into a group of cattle being herded down a two-lane road by real cowboys, who stared at what they must have seen as three crazy hippies. We stopped at General George Armstrong Custer's Battlefield and then Yellowstone National Park, so naïve that we kept mistaking elk for deer. The sheer overstimulation of seeing sites never seen before almost helped me forget my OCD.

My job for the Park Service on the Olympic Peninsula consisted of maintaining and cleaning several large campgrounds spread over a wide area. Each camping area consisted of 30 to 40 camping sites which were filled to near capacity for most of the summer. I was a glorified janitor, cleaning bathrooms and fire pits, clearing trails and paths. At the end of June, I was offered a full-time, year-round position with full benefits with the National Park Service. I was very adept at; hiding any visible symptoms from peers and fellow workers, working hard, requiring little supervision, and I was always helpful to the park visitors. While OCD stayed in the back of my mind, I continued to attend mass every week, conducted by a traveling priest. My brother Pat, Willie and I took an extended trip to San Francisco to visit Uncle Joseph, my godfather, and life was good, with no pressure from school or our work.

My brother and Willie returned to college in August for pre-season football practice. After taking them to the airport, I was forced to change my future: would I stay out west or go home and marry Betsy and finish school? I devoted significant thought and prayer to this question, deciding that Betsy was the most positive aspect of my life. Around Labor Day, I quit my job without notifying my supervisors face-to-face. I left a printed note for them explaining my return to college for the fall semester, but refused to perform this responsibility in person.

That fall in D.C, I was intensely busy and I thrived and was happy, free of OCD episodes. I received a federal educational grant toward my tuition and was accepted into an excellent special education program with 30 other students, all women. I began playing fall baseball for the university squad, while coaching freshman football at my high school. Four evenings a week I was a night watchman and I still tended bar for my good friend, Prep grad Bobby Abbo. As Betsy and I were planning our January wedding, my OCD incidents started to return. As the wedding date approached, I made a confession to a priest, but was troubled afterwards, because it wasn't specific enough regarding my obsessions and behaviors.

Since high school, I have been bothered—after going to and making what I believed was a good confession— by not making a good enough confession. Invariably, I would worry about the validity and sincerity of my most recent confession, and then this OCD pattern would return. I would think, "I did not confess that sexual sin specifically with sufficient detail. I did not tell the priest accurately how many times I thought of sex with a woman, not Betsy." The doubt in my mind would grow and intensify. Then the head tics or other ritualistic behavior began. I might walk back and forth in the garage or backyard and start remembering potential sins that I had forgotten to confess. The conflict sometimes continued for hours.

In this particular confession situation, most of the sexual questions had to do with Betsy, as I worried about having committed mortal sins with her, even though we had never had intercourse before marriage. My anxiety over this issue was reaching the trigger point.

During a fraternity party that fall I attended with Betsy and two baseball teammates, an intoxicated fraternity member made disparaging remarks about my fiancé to her face. I found a sawed off baseball bat, grabbed the guy, and threatened to beat him senseless if he didn't recant. My baseball buddies restrained me, even though the jerk was nearly twice my size. My friends didn't realize I had no intention of hitting the guy. I was bluffing and the situation dissipated, but my anger continued to simmer.

The marital plans came together beautifully, thanks to Betsy and her mom, without much effort on my part. My only major request was that Betsy study religion courses, to become a Catholic before the wedding. She agreed to weekly classes with the pastor of the church where we would be married. Certainly, this demand on Betsy was part of my OCD behavior and it continued after we were married.

Betsy was also confirmed in the Catholic Church and for the next quarter of a century, we strictly followed the rules and tenets of Catholicism. We practiced the rhythm method of birth control and raised our four children in the faith. Our children all attended parochial school, grades K-8, and the two eldest attended Catholic secondary school. As a teacher, I spent ten of my first fifteen years employed in parochial schools. Only after an incident with our third child did Betsy and I begin to question seriously the church's rules and practices. Suffice it to say that our child was brutally bullied for two years while attending a parochial school, and the school's two senior administrators did very little to stop the bullying, refusing to punish those responsible for this atrocious behavior. Our child persevered, primarily because of personal strength and character and the love and support of the family.

From Betsy:

*I truly believe that Jim and I have been here on earth—together—before. How else do you explain my knowing I was going to marry him before ever meeting him? Being with Jim, always felt like we had known each other our entire lives. Everything that's happened in our lives seems to have been "how it is supposed to be," as if it were preordained or some-*

*thing. Getting married was just the next step in our relation-
ship. I knew that Jim had some "hang-ups." Who doesn't? He
basically had saved me as much as I had saved him. He saved
me when I was dealing with my father's alcoholism and I have
saved Jim while he's dealt with OCD. I agreed to convert to
Catholicism because Jim was stronger in his religion than I
was. For me it was an easy decision, especially since we were
going to have children. I felt it was better to raise them together
in one religion, and my parents agreed. There was no conflict
about that, and Catholicism wasn't that much different from
how I was raised as a Presbyterian. I'd been in the choir and
gone to Sunday school, youth group and church every Sunday.
I just wasn't brought up with the "Catholic guilt" that Jim was.*

Betsy and I were married in January of 1972, and enjoyed a
week-long honeymoon in the Pocono Mountains of Pennsylvania. We began our married lives residing in Washington, D.
C.. Betsy found a challenging, well-paying job at GW University Hospital, and we rented a small apartment not far from
the campus. I continued taking a full load of college classes in
special education and working two jobs. Again, staying busy
kept my symptoms somewhat under control, yet having sex
regularly provided me with new avenues to experience OCD
thoughts. I worried about how often we had sex and about
following the rhythm method of not having sex when Betsy
was most likely to become pregnant, as practicing Catholics
were forbidden from using any birth control. Rather than
enjoying sexual activity with my wife, I became obsessed with
the rules of the Catholic Church governing sex in marriage.

We faithfully practiced the rhythm method until our fourth child was born; then Betsy had a tubal ligation procedure.

During our first year of marriage, I once grabbed Betsy and pushed her in the middle of an argument. It was the only time, she has said, that she was actually afraid of me. In that moment, I was experiencing an OCD thought which I could not remove from my mind, and I took my anger and frustration out on her. I never did this again and sought out a counselor to talk with about my anger and obsessive thoughts. This was 1972 and no one had yet diagnosed OCD.

We began regularly seeing a psychiatrist, Dr. D'Agostino, who also happened to be a lawyer, who also happened to be a Jesuit priest. Supposedly, Dr. D'Agostino was one of the leading experts in dealing with someone like me. He was stern, cold, uncaring and lacked any empathy for our dilemma as a newly-married couple.

"Your condition," he told us, "is going to become much worse, before it can become better."

"Well, thanks Doc," I said. "I appreciate your concern, but I am searching for help here. I don't need you telling me how miserable life is going to be. I am already living in pain."

Betsy and I discontinued meeting with Dr. D'Agostino after three or four sessions. Betsy and I both felt negative toward him for years to come.

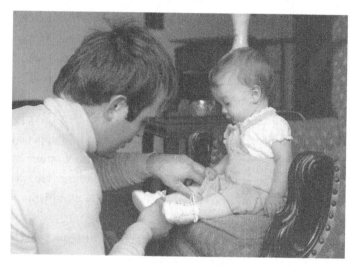

Author and first child Amy
Aurora, CO, 1975

# Chapter VIII

# Moving On

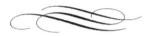

*I*n the spring of 1973, following considerable deliberation, I convinced Betsy we should relocate to Denver, Colorado, as I was struggling almost daily with my OCD thoughts. On a weekend prior to our move west, Betsy had one of her best friends to our apartment for dinner. Following a delicious meal, the three of us drove to the Student Union Building on campus to bowl. While enjoying our bowling, I experienced a sexual thought I could not dismiss and became more and more agitated. I told the girls I had to go home—no explanation, I just had to leave.

I was overwhelmed mentally by attempting to stop thinking about the pretty co-eds bowling a few lanes to our right. The obsessive thoughts were impossible to remove or ignore, and I became more and more frustrated and angry at myself. Betsy knew what was troubling me, but her friend was taken by surprise. Forty-five years later, I can vividly recall walking ahead of them on the sidewalk on campus to our car, visibly distraught, having ruined the evening's fun for all of us. I was embarrassed and ashamed of myself for not being able to control my own thoughts. I felt terrible for Betsy and her dear friend who was also my good friend. I was disgusted by my behavior, and then depressed.

These OCD incidents were becoming more and more regular, and I thought a physical relocation across the country might help. We knew two people in our destination city of Denver; one was my brother Pat and the other my closest friend from high school. Betsy badly missed her mother and cried every day for the first three months. She found an excellent administrative position in her field, and I enrolled at the University of Northern Colorado, hoping to graduate in two years with a degree in education. We began seeing a therapist, a very attentive and concerned psychologist, but he was not successful in helping me with my obsessive thoughts and behaviors.

For the next two years, I was depressed or anxious and angry roughly half of the time. I did well in my college classes, taking eighteen credit hours or more each semester while maintaining a B+ average until graduation in May of 1975. Summers, I worked as a YMCA director of a group of elementary children and became even more adept at hiding or camouflaging my incidents from the counselors and children. Betsy was now a medical secretary for several doctors with large practices. With her mother's assistance, we purchased our first home, which I remodeled and updated. Through all this, I was normal one moment and ready to explode the next.

I returned to punching myself in the face until I looked as if I had been beaten in an alley fight. My eyes became swollen almost shut, with bruises and cuts on my cheeks, nose and forehead. Sometimes, because of my appearance, I skipped school and remained in the house. This went on for more than a year. I knocked holes in the wall, and threw lamps or books or whatever was not too heavy to heave across a room. Away from others, I dented automobiles by kicking them, ruined mirrors and pictures, tossed tools, shovels or rakes. This behavior would continue for years.

In the winter of 1974-'75, Betsy was pregnant and our daughter Amy Marie was born in March, as I began three months of student teaching. We were ecstatic and, being the oldest of eight children, I was experienced with infants and changing diapers, bathing and feeding our baby. I completed undergraduate school in June of 1975, with a major in education and a minor in psychology and a 3.2 GPA. I worked a final summer as an assistant director at a suburban YMCA while looking for a teaching position. In many ways, I seemed normal, at least to outsiders.

Then, early in our daughter's life, my OCD resurfaced with a vengeance. I became obsessed with never touching my daughter's privates—I could not even change her diaper or give her a bath without worrying. I was overwhelmed with making sure this did not happen. I would never have touched her in an immoral manner, yet I worried incessantly about how I changed, bathed and dressed her. I wanted to do my part and be a good, caring, loving father and husband, and somehow I was able to explain all of this to Betsy. I was ashamed for even having such thoughts.

My wife knew instinctively when I experienced difficulties changing our daughter and selflessly took over for me, helping me to stumble through these situations.

From Betsy:

*Jim not changing the children's diapers was never a big deal for me. I knew it bothered him so my doing this eased his pain. He really wasn't around all that much anyway, with teaching and coaching three sports. He'd leave at 7:00 a.m. and most days wouldn't get home until 9:00 at night, when the children were already in bed. On weekends, he either had a game, a tournament or coaches' meetings, so I just took care of this.*

Numerous times Betsy and I discussed how my OCD affected my interaction with our children and how much I regretted not being able to properly care for them. I remain sickened by all the precious moments with our four children I lost being distracted by obsessions and compulsions—one of the saddest parts of my secret life and my public life.

What is most disturbing is that my OCD, when caring for our infants, never diminished. Betsy and I parented three more children and I was never able comfortably to help with them as a father should. The identical obsessions have plagued me with our three grandchildren, who are now in elementary and middle school. What a disheartening chain of events I was unable to change!

Throughout the summer following my college graduation, I applied for dozens of teaching and coaching positions. I was 26, with a degree in education, with three years of coaching high school football, and three years as a youth program director. Despite all of my experience, I wasn't able to secure a full-time teaching position. I signed up to substitute teach, but after several negative experiences, including witnessing a fight between two high school upperclassmen, I looked elsewhere for employment. Eventually, I answered an ad for United Parcel Service and became a UPS delivery driver and member of the Teamsters Union. The hours, compensation and benefits were excellent, but I kept thinking that I had not spent seven years in college to drive a truck and drop off packages.

My OCD soon impacted my new job. In the 1970's, UPS drivers were required to obtain real signatures from almost every patron on their routes, as these documents proving delivery were turned in each evening. When I entered the name and address for each package, my mind told me that I could not end writing with the tip of a letter pointing toward the privates of my female customer or a possible bystander—a grievous sin. To compensate, I had to draw additional lines and circles on my signature records, not appreciated by my supervisor or his bosses, the sheets looking as if I had purposely doodled on my official paperwork. When asked to discontinue this practice by my supervisor, I could not explain my unorthodox behavior. I kept the job for eight months, but this obsession never fully stopped.

In late spring of 1976, I resigned from UPS, after taking and passing the preliminary written test and background check for applying to the United States Secret Service, hiring for the upcoming presidential election. Looking back, I should have realized the Secret Service would never have hired me because of my 4F Selective Service status. After passing initial testing and background checks, the Secret Service quickly informed me that they had met their quota for new agents.

I found a position as a full-time teacher, coach and dormitory proctor at Bullis Prep School back in Washington. My wife and I and our one-year old daughter moved to D.C, where Betsy secured a good government position, and we purchased a townhouse in the country. I led the varsity soccer team to the school's first-ever IAC League Championship, organized and started a Varsity Club Organization for athletes and began a comprehensive weight training program for all students while teaching a full schedule of physical education classes.

Despite my success and enjoyment from teaching and mentoring young students, I could not escape OCD. During the championship season, I called in sick several days in a row because I was experiencing obsessive thoughts, leading to serious depression. Betsy and I talked often about my minimal salary and the high cost of living in D.C., as well as the pressure we felt living close to our families.

There was, to be sure, no love lost between my father and my mother-in-law, Betty Lingo. To say they hated one another is too harsh, but they disagreed on many of life's important issues: religion, politics, morals, etc. Our two families lived a block apart at the Jersey shore, but might as well have been in different countries for all they had in common. As often happens, my father and mother-in-law were very alike in some ways: my father could be arrogant and haughty, Betty very sure of herself and opinionated, not good attributes in the eyes of many Italian males. Dad often acted superior to others, while Betty took grief from no one, having fought to maintain her family in the face of her husband's alcoholism. The Juliana's and Lingo's remained civil with one another mostly out of respect for their children. None of these relatives had any inkling of what Betsy and I lived with every day and we felt more comfortable living away from all of them.

In the spring of 1977, I went to a Catholic church to offer a very sincere and good confession for mortal sins in recent years. I did this in anticipation of returning to Colorado and beginning anew my professional teaching and coaching career. Before moving west, I inquired into a one-year internship and practice teaching in an exclusive private school tailored to children with special education needs. I secured two temporary jobs: one as a National Park Service Ranger in the summer and the other a two-year, full-time, graduate assistantship in adaptive physical education for my master's degree. The offer came from one of the state's largest universities, Colorado State, and while the compensation wasn't much, I had been selected from more than 100 other applicants. The opportunity looked great, but then…

Later that spring of 1977, Betsy became pregnant with our second child, and I turned down the graduate assistant position; I was afraid of my OCD ruining my assistantship. Instead I took the job as a special education intern teacher at the private school. My life-long career in teaching and coaching was about to commence in earnest once again, but would my undiagnosed OCD allow us to be happily married, good parents and successful in our careers?

From Betsy:

*When the children were small and I could sense that "things" were bothering Jim, I would remove them from the situation or divert their attention away from him. At times he would seem to do crazy things, but they never questioned them. For me, having four children in five years made a lot of that period of my life a blur. Not only was I raising them, with Jim away most of the time coaching, but I was also running our family-owned, dry cleaning business that the children eventually came to help and run.*

*Jim was also really good at hiding his OCD. I'm not sure how the children felt, but I pretty much always knew when he was dealing with his OCD, because I could see him staring off into space. I could see his lips moving as he was repeating things over and over in his mind. Of course, you couldn't hide when he would hit a wall or hit his head with his fists, but he did that when the children weren't around.*

*I can't remember an actual time when we told the children about Jim having OCD. When they were little, they always knew there was something odd about Dad at times, but they never questioned his unusual behavior. As they became older, they seemed to be more aware, but we knew very little about OCD and just figured that was how Dad was.*

*"I wonder how Dad will be when he gets home," they sometimes said, because you never knew which "Dad" you were going to get when he walked through the door. He was either dealing with an obsession or had gotten it under control by the time he arrived home. If he seemed in a bad mood, the children*

*disappeared to do their own activities.*

*As time went on and OCD became a something we could "name," the children wanted to know more and we discussed it. Of course, now they know he has OCD and will often laugh about it or talk about having symptoms of their own— but not to the degree Jim has it. Our three girls are teachers and their obsession with organization parallels OCD, but nothing too alarming.*

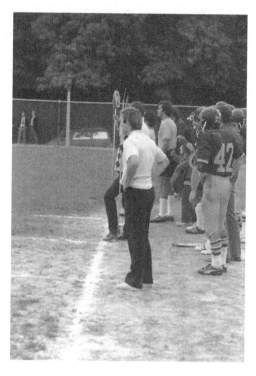

Author—Coaching Football
Washington, D. C., 1976

# Chapter IX

# Teaching

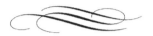

*I*t is important to understand why I chose teaching as a profession and how OCD significantly affected every aspect of my professional life, constantly interfering with my daily schedule. I occasionally contemplate how much more I might have accomplished as a teacher and mentor without this burden.

Watching youngsters grow and improve was very satisfying to me. I enjoyed being a mentor and motivator and felt that by teaching I could repay all the wonderful instructors who shaped my life and simultaneously give back for how much I had received. As my career evolved, I came to believe that teaching was a personal, higher calling, a vocation more than simply an occupation, an attempt to perform good works for others. I have repeatedly faced negative school environments with virtually no discipline, low academic achievement, little success in athletics and dysfunctional leadership. Despite this, I have always tried to have a nurturing influence on students and athletes.

I believe that being battered by OCD has provided me with a personal toughness, a fierce determination to not give in or give up. I have never taken drugs or tried to commit suicide. Why I have not experienced these activities strikes me as a sort of miracle. More than anything, I consider myself a survivor. I have persevered through a very trying time in high school and prep school, decades of despondence over OCD, prostate cancer at sixty, the loss of hearing in one ear, and the daily struggle with my secret life since age ten. Each of these obstacles has made me stronger. As a teacher and coach, I used my experiences to show young people that with hard work, dedication, and perseverance, they too could overcome what life throws at them, as it kept throwing new challenges at me.

In my late twenties and early thirties, I endured multiple, lengthy periods when OCD would not allow me to read anything: a book, newspaper or magazine. Very often, this behavior occurred as I was studying for undergraduate and then graduate school classes or when reading for pleasure, a most favorite and cherished pastime.

As I was studying to take my comprehensive examination to finish my master's degree and faced with preparing a series of extensive essay responses, I was unable to read and study. When I tried to read, certain words caused me to think sexual or perverse thoughts, and I could not finish a single page of text. No matter what I did to eliminate the thoughts— shaking my head, closing my eyes, whispering "no" to myself, pausing for a moment or saying a silent prayer—it didn't stop my graphic thoughts. Miraculously, during the four-hour long master's examination, I answered a required three of the five essay questions sufficiently to pass on my first attempt. Luck, native intelligence or divine intervention—I cannot explain my good fortune.

Indirectly because of OCD, I had trouble remaining in the same teaching position for more than a few years. I would initially impress other instructors and students with my organizational and motivational skills, but soon I wanted to move on. I was quite capable of professionally resolving the difficult issues with students, but much less so with fellow teachers whom I often saw as lazy or incompetent. I repeatedly had serious problems with administrators whom I believed cared more about their position than the welfare of their students and school. Once again, my problems with authority and its misuse and abuse had re-emerged.

I believe strongly in fairness and justice, and I am unafraid of voicing my concerns despite possible negative consequences. In situation after situation, I have butted heads with someone in a well-placed position above me. After losing respect for a principal or administrator, I would often strongly confront them on an issue and this inevitably cost me my job. As I have said, I do not think OCD caused my problems with authority, but OCD left me angry, frustrated, and vulnerable to conflict that made me seek new employment.

OCD was always just under the surface, waiting to erupt.

Years ago I was driving to see my therapist in Denver and unknowingly made an illegal U-turn on a corner by his office. As I slowly drove back up the block toward the hospital and parallel parked, I passed two police officers making a house-call. Early for my appointment, I pulled out a textbook and tried to study for a graduate class, when I was suddenly interrupted by a severely obsessive thought, causing me to begin a ritualistic compulsion to try to remove the unwanted thought.

I was deeply involved in the compulsion when the police drove up beside my car. The two officers stepped from their cruiser and in my agitated state I muttered to myself, "Shit, what do these assholes want?" This attitude came as a result of the obsession/compulsion, not from disrespect for the police.

Just to be clear, this is not who I am. My father was an FBI special agent and I am pro-police, but I was not myself. Getting out of the car, I used the F-word and demanded an explanation for being questioned. One officer cuffed me, lifting me off of my feet by my wrists and pushing me onto the roof of my car. I knew I was in trouble and did not resist at all. I was under arrest for the first time ever—on a traffic violation, the illegal U-turn. After I spent several hours in jail, Betsy bailed me out. Weeks later, I had to undergo surgery on my elbow; while being hoisted up by my wrists, the officer had severely damaged the ulnar nerve in my left elbow. I later filed an excessive force complaint against the police department, but to no avail.

Lesson One: Do not lose your temper with the cops. Lesson Two: Obsessive compulsive disorder may contribute to more serious problems and consequences.

I have always believed that my arrest was caused by my OCD symptoms. I realized that I had been disrespectful to the police—my obsession and compulsion in response to an unwanted thought had caused me to become angry at them and this troubled me greatly. Without OCD, I would have been polite and honest with them, yet there I was in hand-cuffs, being arrested with a serious injury to my arm, which would later require major surgery. It was one more manifestation of how a phobia could bring my family and me mental, physical, emotional and financial harm. OCD symptoms can immediately take over one's life and this is exacerbated in precarious situations.

Not long after this incident, I was diagnosed by my psychiatrist, Dr. Baucum, as dealing with a chemical imbalance in my brain, caused by the neurotransmitter serotonin. Now, for the first time ever, I heard the term Obsessive Compulsive Disorder. At last, the demon had a name. It was 1984, and new information concerning brain disorders and dysfunctions was being uncovered frequently by medical researchers.

With Dr. Baucum in charge of my treatment, I began cognitive behavior therapy (CBT) and taking medication—serotonin re-uptake inhibitors (SRIs) –and this continued for twenty years, until he retired. For much of the first two decades of my educational career, I saw Dr. Baucum once a month. In addition to every other problem I was combating, this therapy was a significant financial burden on Betsy's and my marriage and family.

Over the past 34 years, I have been prescribed a host of medications: Anafranil, Louvox, Zoloft, Prozac, and then Prozac with Buspar, Lexepro, Celexa, and currently Cymbalta, along with one drug not sanctioned by the USFDA, which Dr. Baucum had obtained legally from Canada.

I was eager to try any new drug as it came on the market, if he thought it might be helpful. Some of the drugs left me edgy and jittery, so I stopped taking them. Prozac, which I was on the longest, caused me to become drowsy. At school, I often fell asleep in my office chair between classes or during free periods. This sleep was mostly induced by depression and by medications or by exhaustion—the mental and physical fatigue from trying to function with OCD.

In one therapy, Dr. Baucum put rubber bands around my wrists and every time I developed an obsessive thought, I would snap the tight band against my skin to stop it from becoming repetitive. This was not very effective so we graduated to electro-shock therapy. Desperate for help, I agreed to try it. I have never been tortured in military conflict, but 30 years after this experience I can say that enduring just one session of this treatment conjures in my imagination that level of agony. I have a fairly high threshold for pain, but having an electrode connected to my forefinger and knowing I was going to be hit with an electrical charge strong enough to cause my hand to jump off the chair arm and almost make me urinate, was torture enough. I was in this procedure for about 20 minutes and when it ended and I walked out to my car, I had to stand still and calm myself to keep from shaking or vomiting. Electro-shock therapy had no noticeable effect on lessening my obsessions or compulsions and we never attempted this again.

When my OCD was at its strongest, the most important time in combating it was right as the obsession (thought) first entered my brain. If I could block it at the very start, I could occasionally stop the thought before reverting to ritualistic compulsions intended to push it out of my mind. Sometimes, I shook my head to try to remove the unwanted thought– or imagined a positive place by using a familiar word, like baseball. If an unwanted thought came into my mind, and I could not immediately stop or block it, I was usually doomed to falling back into ritualistic compulsions. Stopping the thought quickly was far more effective than attempting to remove it through a compulsion.

The anger, aggression and violence I experienced from trying to cope with OCD were most often initiated by my inability to remove an embedded thought. My frustration multiplied to the point where it turned into anger and sometimes violence ensued, followed by severe despair, depression and thoughts of suicide. It happened over and over again and my "OCD Stare," as some labeled my expression when in this state, originated from this as well: a glazed-over look reflecting bewilderment, suffocation, demoralization and at a complete loss for answers.

I do not like being confrontational and take no enjoyment from losing my temper, but OCD often adversely affected the way I acted with the people I most loved—my family and friends. In public or on the job, I regularly behaved in ways I would never have dreamed of acting, and to this day I regret many of my actions.

During these years, my desperation was deepening. My family saw me:

- Teaching and coaching in nine different schools during a twenty-two year time period and not being content for long with any of my professional situations.

- Getting fired from three head football positions, not for poor coaching performance, but for disagreeing with administrators on philosophy, policy and procedures.

- Alienating numerous educational peers and friends while holding them, especially administrators, to high standards of excellence and performance.

- Spending nineteen months unemployed or underemployed due to changing jobs so often.

- Discontinuing the practice of my Catholic faith after one of our children was brutally bullied in his parochial school for two years.

- Repeatedly disagreeing with my parents, especially with my father, on every issue imaginable.

- Causing my wife and children unwarranted stress and worry.

As the children were growing up, I perfected the art of disguise and deception, hiding my OCD from them until they were mature enough to understand that their father possessed severe problems. I tried to deal with my rituals away from their sight by going into the garage or bathroom or outside at night. In public, if I could gather enough self-control, I would hold off until in the privacy of home.

When the children were quite young, I once endured a series of obsessions over several hours, becoming more and more angry and frustrated, physically and emotionally exhausted. Finally, I took a kitchen knife and—away from everyone—stabbed the back of an upholstered, living room chair, a gift from my parents, leaving a huge hole in its back. Days later when preparing to throw the chair out, I noticed that our youngest daughter, five or six at the time, had attempted to repair the hole by covering it with duct tape. Only a vicious disorder would compel a loving father to commit such an unnatural act.

Another ritual that occurred hundreds, if not thousands, of times came when I was building a wooden deck on the back of our home and again as I was doing this for a friend. In both instances, our only son Jimmy, who was around twelve, was helping me. I was screwing some boards to the joists with an electric drill and the act reminded me of sexual intercourse. The obsession kept repeating itself and strengthening within my mind, as I became more upset and angry—yelling at my son, demanding that he perform supportive tasks beyond his capabilities. My heart rate rose and I perspired heavily, as I proceeded from obsessive thoughts to verbal explosions to forcing myself to drive the screw perfectly straight to satisfy the compulsion. I could not do it perfectly, so I would start over by removing the screw and repeating the entire process with a new screw. I did this until satisfied that each screw was perfectly straight and I could stop the obsessing about it.

Throughout all of this, my son and I both grew more stressed, distraught and at odds with one other. After fifteen or twenty minutes, I gathered myself and regained control, but not before despair came over me, along with the dissolution of any joy and happiness from working with my son. His mood was ruined as well. A terrible feeling of disappointment and loss replaced my love and pride for him, and he has told me that he felt something similar for me. We lost countless opportunities for good times together throughout his youth. I hate OCD for ruining these special opportunities with my son.

On another occasion, I was standing in the middle of our high school football team's pregame warm-ups. I was mentally engrossed with dispelling an obsession when the opposing head coach approached and earnestly thanked me for a condolence letter I had sent him regarding his mother's death. He eventually had to hit me on the shoulder to bring me out of my trance, but I was still unable to be fully present with him, generating more frustration and anger. I remember thinking in that moment that if OCD had been a person, I would have torn its throat out with my bare hands.

Every few years, I would try a new medication, but even when the new drug diminished my edginess and anxiety, the obsessions and compulsions continued unabated. Would I ever experience any genuine relief from OCD? Only time would tell.

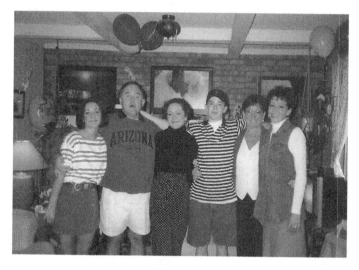

L-R: Stephanie, Jim, Amy, Jimmy, Betsy, Laura
Littleton, CO, mid 90's

# Chapter X

# Silence and Suffering

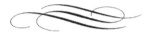

*B*efore retiring in 1999, Dr. Baucum recommended a successful psychiatrist, Dr. Lyons, who specialized in treating adolescents and young adults. When first conferring with Dr. Lyons, I was 51 and liked him immediately. We had much in common, as he was an easterner, a sports buff, a family man and close to my age. Twenty years later he is still my primary care provider and manages my OCD medication.

After leaving the Colorado School of Mines where I had taught and coached for two years, I secured another teaching position in an alternative education high school, a last-chance opportunity for students expelled from a school or multiple schools. Without changing their ways, these students were destined for reform school or prison. Our alternative school accepted those who had been in reform school or incarcerated and were attempting to get back into a regular high school. I was excited to start my new job. My salary was higher than I had received in 22 years of teaching, and I was surrounded by dedicated, hard-working professionals.

For me, the 21st century was starting off well, with a new psychiatrist, a new school and a new football coaching situation. Teaching in any type of alternative environment is challenging, and good discipline and strict organization are required for any significant level of success. The principal who hired me was soon promoted and the educator who took over had no experience in alternative education. She had spent the majority of her career in curriculum development—about as far from her new role as one could get. I liked her, but she lacked practical experience in the classroom when it came to disciplining unruly students.

From Betsy:

*Jim was so good at his profession. Even though he didn't make a lot of money, his passion lay in teaching and coaching. No matter in what school he taught and coached, he was always the most popular teacher and/or coach. He had that ability to be strict, yet respected and loved all at the same time. Even to this day he has students that we see socially, 40 years later.*

*Jim did move around from school to school, but we decided to stay in Littleton and not uproot the children. We are still in the same house 30 years later. Jim has seen many doctors to cure him of this awful disease. How he is still alive to this day amazes me. Only his will to live and overcome OCD and his fortitude have enabled him to get this far. If it had been me, I'd have put a gun to my head years ago.*

Immediately, I felt uncomfortable working with the new principal's liberal philosophy of education. My anxiety level was soon high, but so was my desire to perform well. Many of the students were angry, rebellious and confrontational, but the new principal's views suggested the student is always right and the teacher is always wrong. The daily opportunity for conflict increased my anxiety and contributed to my frustration when I began experiencing OCD obsessions. I was as angry as the students and things would only get worse.

I was coaching at East High School and had befriended a football player arrested for shoplifting. I agreed to testify on his behalf, went to the courthouse, and spoke about his good character in an effort to keep him out of jail. Before leaving school that morning, I told the school secretary where I was going and how long I'd be there. Later, the principal excoriated me for leaving school and for trying to help this young man—not what I wanted in my new job.

In the early 2000's, I began researching my attitude toward those in authority, hoping to find a hospital or university engaged in uncovering what causes OCD. The National Institutes of Health (NIH) in Bethesda, Maryland, was engaged in research to isolate the familial gene behind OCD. I convinced my sister, two brothers, a paternal uncle, my uncle's son, and his daughter to participate in the study with me, which included answering a multitude of personal and medical questions, along with providing an oral swab. We received a minimal amount of compensation for our involvement, which initiated some frank and productive dialogue among family members.

Despite living 2,000 miles apart, my youngest brother and I have carried on a meaningful discourse on how OCD affects us and how certain medications have significantly diminished major symptoms—most especially Lexapro. Our brothers and sister also display periodic OCD obsessions and compulsions, but I have never felt comfortable engaging them in this subject. Admitting that one suffers from a lifelong mental illness is not something many people want to divulge to relatives and friends.

In my family, the idea that our father was OCD-impaired was usually handled as a joke, something to be laughed at. This was incredibly ignorant on our part, as I strongly believe that problems of this nature can never be solved unless confronted head on. Just as my mother's alcoholism was ignored, our family's OCD was avoided to eliminate discomfort and embarrassment; suggesting family members seek treatment might have offended them. At my advanced age, I have chosen to speak out and address the issues surrounding OCD, doing everything I can to make life easier and more productive for anyone who suffers from OCD.

I never considered asking my father to join in the OCD study yet he was the most obvious person in our family suffering from it. I have never told any employer about my OCD, considering this to be my problem and my problem alone. I have tried as hard as possible to hide this from those with whom I have worked. OCD has never been debilitating enough to affect definitively my teaching or coaching or mentoring students.

Individuals of my father's generation, especially males, never spoke about issues like mental health or addictions. Some members of my family still will not discuss OCD, a major mistake in my experience; one cannot defeat the disorder without first acknowledging he/she suffers from it. The NIH had also told members of its OCD study group that we wouldn't receive any news on the results of the genetic testing, so I don't know if a familial gene for OCD was ever isolated. Once again, Betsy and I were left with trying to penetrate this mystery on our own.

Since 2000, I have taken various new medications to relieve my symptoms. My youngest brother has used Lexapro in his struggle with OCD, and my brother Robert says the drug has significantly helped him. For years I took it as well and it left me much calmer. My anxiety level was lower and I was less apt to get angry or emotional when dealing with obsessions or compulsions. It didn't make me drowsy or sleepy.

But problems remained.

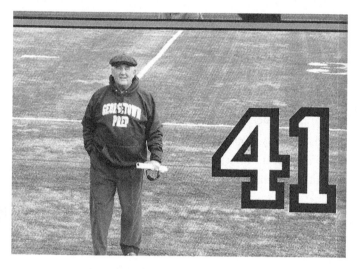

Author at Georgetown Preparatory School
Washington, D. C., November, 2010

# Chapter XI

# Completing My Teaching Career

*A*t the end of my first year teaching at the alternative high school in Denver Public Schools, the principal made me sign an agreement: to be rehired for the following year, I would have to complete and pass an Anger Management Class over summer break. The psychologist who gave the class questioned why I was taking the class. She remarked, "You do not appear to me to require anger management. There certainly are many teachers in today's classrooms that could benefit from anger management, since there is basically no discipline in the majority of schools. But you seem above all that." I passed the course, and returned to the alternative school the following school year, still experiencing 25-30 OCD incidents a day, but taking Lexapro to help control my anger and frustration.

During 2001-2002, I faced two challenging situations. First, a young man I was tutoring free of charge after school, made a motion as if he were going to stab me with a pencil while I was tutoring him. I gripped his shirt collar and forced him into the dean's office. I found out later that the boy's mother told the principal that she had forgotten to give her son his anti-psychotic medication that morning. The second incident came at an all-school assembly when a new student (a street gang member) continued to make loud negative comments to a guest drama group from another school. After numerous requests by several teachers and an administrator to behave, I grabbed the young man's ear and led him into an alcove, where I had him sit quietly until the performance was over. The principal accompanied the 6' 1", 200-pound student upstairs and queried him. He told her that he wanted to speak with me, and we went into my classroom and closed the door, facing down one another, two feet apart. He reached out his hand to shake mine and I took it.

"Hey, man," he said, "you and I are okay. I was acting like an ass down there and you were the only adult to stand up to me. We're cool."

He walked quietly out of my room.

In both situations, I used more physical force than acceptable today. I was frustrated and should have utilized more appropriate behavior. Yet I was the only teacher or administrator to hold the students accountable. At the end of that year, I was forced by the principal to transfer out of the alternative school. I applied and received an eighth grade teaching position in a middle school.

I had reached the bottom of the barrel, and the beginning of the end of my teaching career. I was 54 with a master's degree, plus 50 additional graduate hours. Betsy and I had two children attending college and another daughter who would be married in the summer of 2002, our first child to marry. When I should have been at the peak of my teaching and coaching career, I was flailing, simply trying to survive, in large part because of OCD. After almost 25 years of teaching and thirty years of coaching, I remained unable to control my OCD symptoms on the job.

The more that administrators coddled students and refused to bring belligerent ones to account, the more angry and frustrated I became with those in authority. The more I tried to adjust to the new status quo in teaching environments, the worse my OCD became. My symptoms, my age and my personal commitment to excellence and traditional values were all unraveling my career. I had reached a juncture where I was losing the physical and emotional strength and the desire to continue battling OCD.

At the new middle school, I discovered that I was slated to teach sixth graders, not the eighth graders I had been promised by the principal in the spring when I signed my contract. So happy to have any teaching position, I uncharacteristically did not protest to the principal about my change in assignment. I optimistically began teaching sixth graders as part of a team with four females, three of them the same age as our two oldest daughters. I deferred to them and assumed a very minor role within the team. The ladies appreciated me as an effective, experienced teacher, and I needed their support and assistance, as sixth graders are a challenge to organize, teach and discipline. My last class of the day that year had 36 students, twelve of whom had Individualized Educational Plans and a myriad of educational, discipline or emotional problems, a very difficult situation.

At work, I was constantly fighting off obsessions and

compulsions and began to develop chest pains over time, which gradually intensified. One day I notified the office to contact my wife, who picked me up and drove me to the hospital. Following an intensive medical exam, I was found to be in good health, but suffering from stress. After lengthy discussions with Betsy and my primary care physician, I asked that he write a letter recommending I not return to school for the last six weeks of the year, and he wholeheartedly agreed.

I felt utterly overwhelmed. The combination of stress at school and OCD had defeated me. After leaving my teaching position, my obsessions and compulsions increased in frequency and severity—because I had much more free time to engage in these activities. My old pattern was back in play: I would secure a job and begin a new teaching and coaching position, but within a couple of years, I would be searching for work once again. My final two years as a classroom teacher took place from 2003 through 2005, exactly thirty years after earning my undergraduate degree. I accepted a job as a seventh grade social studies teacher and the head varsity football coach for a high school team that hadn't won a game in two seasons. I was named the high school head varsity baseball coach as well, when dealing with around 25-30 OCD incidents per day.

The faculty at the middle school was relatively young, the first-year principal a seasoned teacher in her late thirties. I became a kind of unofficial mentor to her and some of the other instructors. Being treated with respect and appreciation by my peers made me feel better than I had felt while teaching in years. Being seen as a father figure by my fellow teachers took away much of my stress, which in turn made me stronger vis-à-vis my OCD. With the exception of not being able to win any football games, everything else at school was good: the students, parents, other teachers, and principal were supportive and kind.

The school year progressed well through the fall and winter quarters, and I maintained excellent rapport with the high school principal. He and I were both new to the district, and shared many common values and ideas. My stress level was manageable; my OCD incidents fewer and more easily dismissed. Betsy and I hosted a Christmas party attended by the junior high faculty, the principal and several parents. I was successfully hiding from my peers and co-workers any of the signs of struggling with OCD. Following the holidays, I requested that my high school building keys be returned to me, so I could run the off-season, weight-training sessions after school for the football players at the high school building, a common practice for head football coaches. The athletic director, who was the football coach I had replaced and the superintendent refused my request, due to school policy regarding keys. Additional archaic district rules and procedures were used to curtail my success in rebuilding the football and baseball programs.

The pattern of not interacting appropriately with my superiors—the AD and superintendent—arose again. The AD had refused to pay me my $3,000 salary for coaching football, because I had not returned my keys to him first after the season ended. I challenged the AD in front of the principal in the AD's office.

"If you ever refuse to pay me a check I have already earned," I said to the AD, "because I haven't turned in my school keys, you will have a serious problem with me. You have no right to treat my family and me that way!"

The seventh school and the seventh instance where I could not work successfully and professionally with individuals in power and authority. Was I failing because I wanted to fail? Or because of my misplaced set of personal values? Were my failures due to anger, aggressiveness, my disdain for authority figures, and even my profession? Were my failures because of the OCD influences that had never abated? Or were they the result of my immaturity, pettiness and insecurity?

I left this school in the spring of 2005, under the excuse of a RIFT procedure: Reduction In Force Transfer, after the two highest-paid teachers in the middle school, me included, who were very productive, caring and well-liked instructors, were forced to look for employment in another school district because of district cutbacks. My career in education was officially finished.

From Betsy:

*When Jim left teaching, I was glad and relieved, because it was taking such an emotional toll on him. The kids he coached and taught weren't the same as before, especially those in the last five years of his career. Actually, there wasn't much teaching going on. At Emerson Street School, he had high school kids who'd been kicked out of every school they'd enrolled in. The next stop after Emerson was jail, so it was a full day of dealing with belligerent, angry teenagers. Not much fun and a lot of babysitting. At Grant Middle School, he had 39 sixth graders in one class, eleven of them special education students, and no aide to assist him. All he could do was try to keep order. His passion for dealing with the educational system, for the sake of children, was gone. The only thing he really missed was coaching, which is why he still helps out with "scouting" and giving pep talks to football players.*

Sometime in my past, a psychologist or psychiatrist told me that my OCD symptoms would probably diminish with age, but that wasn't the case. My OCD symptoms have fluctuated in intensity over different periods during my life, ranging from moderate to bad to severe to debilitating. My typical obsessions fall into four categories: 1) Intrusive random sexual thoughts and/or urges; 2) Scrupulosity, which is excessive religious moral doubt and indecision; 3) Forbidden thoughts; 4) The need to tell, ask and confess to someone. The most common compulsions beside my head tics and the feeling of pins in my eyes are as follows: 1) Confessing to my mom as a child and worrying constantly about committing a particular mortal sin and being damned to hell for eternity; or having to attend confession in church and convincing myself I had not committed a mortal sin, but then having the same thought return and repeating the entire sequence; 2) Repetitive praying and rethinking the act of possibly sinning over and over to determine if I did or did not actually commit a sin, which could take minutes, hours or days; 3) Forcing of a forbidden thought from my mind, sexual or otherwise, and then staring at a particular spot on the wall or ceiling or floor for seconds or minutes to reassure myself that I had waited a sufficient time before "I can go on with my life as usual," often repeating this phrase to end the compulsion; 4) Believing I must confess to mortal sins from years or decades ago, which I may or may not have already confessed to—or I will go to hell when I die.

Staring at a spot on the wall or the ceiling or at another object while trying to convince my brain that I was not a sinner, often kept me from going crazy and losing my temper or destroying something around me. Some other ritualistic compulsions were shaking my head side to side, praying the same prayer over and over again, chanting words to myself, sleeping for lengthy periods of time or swearing profusely at God. There are many more.

I have also forced myself to engage in random compulsions: hand washing, re-combing my hair, rituals in how I get dressed, how I end my writing on a page and not allowing the final pen or pencil mark to point toward privates, not stepping on cracks in the sidewalk, sitting so my private parts do not point toward a woman's privates, and not allowing a dog to walk over and touch my privates. A common recurring obsession is that whenever I attempt to calm myself by breathing deeply and thinking about a special place, I must not exhale onto myself, because that would be committing a serious sin. Since Dr. Gallagher taught me this relaxation technique several years ago, I have this compulsion every time I try the breathing technique.

Even though I have not been a strict, practicing Catholic

for nearly 25 years, and even though I made a pact with Dr. Gallagher over three years ago not to attend church or go to confession or pray regularly, my Catholic upbringing and many years of practicing my faith continued to influence my obsessions and compulsions on a daily basis.

A singular moment in my life came in June 2006 after my mother, Bette, underwent life-saving, emergency surgery for a ruptured intestine. Her surgeons wondered if she could survive, so I rushed back to New Jersey. For the quarter century before this, she had repeated to her husband and children, one of them a licensed funeral director and accomplished mortician, "Never, ever, do I want to be placed on a respirator or life-support system!"

I flew into south Jersey early on a Friday morning and rushed to the hospital to find my mother gravely ill. Since learning of her condition, I had been completely unhampered by any OCD obsessions or compulsions. Other than Betsy, my mother was the only woman with whom I had ever felt comfortable and at ease. Lying in bed, surrounded by my father and two of my siblings, I realized that mother was not only conscious, but very, very angry, visibly shaken and distraught.

As I bent over and kissed her, she attempted to communicate with me through her breathing mask, but I could not decipher her words. A nurse came in and told my dad the surgeon wished to speak to him. He left and my sister and youngest brother followed him out of the room. I grabbed my mother's hand.

"Mother," I said, "what do you want me to do?"

With both hands, she reached for the mask, but was too weak to remove it.

"Off the mask, off the mask," she repeated

She rolled her head side to side. "No. No mask."

"Mom, you were always my best friend. You know that, don't you? I love you Mom."

"I know, I know. No mask," she mumbled once again.

"I'll get it removed as soon as we can. I promise you," I said, as the family re-entered my mom's room.

My father, highly distressed, returned to his chair against the wall. My sister tried to say something comforting to my mother, but was quickly rebuffed. I realized that when I had first entered the room, I had interrupted my mother severely reprimanding all of them for allowing her to have been placed on a respirator. I walked over to her to say goodbye and tell her again that I loved her. I never spoke to her again and left the room thinking this was no way to die—so angry at my family.

That afternoon, my sister and two youngest brothers met on the boardwalk in Ocean City, N.J., one of the most visited tourist attractions in town. The raised wooden walkway, extending more than a mile along the beach, is where the daily high tide reaches its peak. The boardwalk is lined with clothing stores, souvenir shops, restaurants, amusement rides and movie houses. Our family had been walking these "boards" for decades. Betsy and I have two boardwalk paintings hanging in our home. I had asked for this get-together to tell my siblings we needed to convince our father to have the physicians remove Mom's respirator. They agreed and we called our brother Pat in Colorado, who concurred.

"Aren't mother's wishes," I said to Pat, "what's most important here?"

"Yes, they are," Pat replied, "but good luck getting Dad to go along with what you're proposing. He won't give in."

That night, four siblings and my father and I had a late meal together at our parents' home on the water. A couple of my siblings drank too much and Dad had a little wine. I drank nothing and was relieved that through the day, no OCD obsessions or compulsions had entered my mind. Dinner was interrupted by a call from mother's surgeon, providing Dad with an update on her condition; she was stable and showing slight improvement.

"Dad," I said, "don't you think it's time to discuss removing Mom from the respirator? She is mad and wants off the machine—like right now!"

Without so much as a pause, he responded, "The doctors will decide when mom gets off the machine. That is their call."

"But she's miserable. You can see it in her face. We have all talked and everyone agrees that mother never wanted to be on a respirator. She has been telling us that for the last twenty-five years. We can't allow her to lay in anguish and pain indefinitely."

In the same somber, unemotional voice, Dad responded, "The doctors know best. End of discussion."

"So, are we just supposed to sit around here while mother suffers in the hospital? The doctors work for us. I'll call her doctor right now and tell him that we, her family, want her off the respirator. If you don't want to phone them, I will."

He stared at me defiantly and snapped, "It's not your call."

"She's my mother and does not deserve this! You're wrong not to do anything. This is bullshit!"

I stood and approached him. My mortician brother grabbed me from behind and locked my arms behind my back. My sister and another brother yelled at me to get out of the house. Our youngest brother quietly moved beside me, gently took my arm and suggested we leave. At that moment, I felt nothing but disdain and disgust for my father for displaying no compassion or sympathy toward my mother, acting like some kind of monarch with supreme power over his subjects. What kept me from breaking away from my brothers and beating him senseless was my sense of pity for him. Here was an old man—with all his authority and money—absolutely powerless to take charge of an unfortunate situation and display his love for our mother. All I wanted was for him to make a phone call demanding they take mother off of the respirator and let her live or die on her own terms, her express wish over so many years.

I turned away from Dad and followed my youngest brother out of the house. Then I pivoted around and stared at my father, who looked worn and old. I yelled at him, in words I won't repeat, that he was terribly wrong, terribly unsympathetic, and a poor excuse for a husband. I continued screaming at him from the street.

The next day, my brother and I stopped by the hospital on our way to Rob's home in Philadelphia. I told him to go in to see Mom alone, as I couldn't bring myself to tell her she would remain on the respirator. Finally, two days later, the doctors removed her from the respirator and she breathed normally without it, improving noticeably until the physicians thought they might release her to go home with a colostomy bag later in the week. Then Betsy and I received a call back in Denver about 1 pm Monday afternoon. After seemingly making a recovery, mother's system began to shut down and she died in the early afternoon, without distress, peacefully. I couldn't help thinking how she had loved and nurtured me so wonderfully when I was a baby and young boy, just starting to live with OCD. It puzzled me that when she was dying I had no OCD symptoms, none at all, unheard of at this juncture in my life.

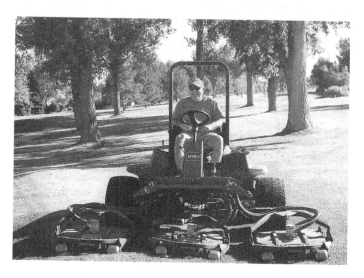

Author
Columbine Country Club
Littleton, CO, 2009

# Chapter XII

# Post-Teaching Era

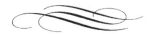

*A*fter regrettably saying farewell to my teaching career in 2005, I turned in a challenging, and dissimilar direction, initiated during the summer between my last two years in education. For the past fifteen years, golf course management, basically cutting and caring for grass, has become my personal mantra. I have not gotten wealthy doing this, but the quality and value of my daily existence has improved considerably. I have had stability in my work situation and with Betsy and my residing in the same suburban, middle class neighborhood for the past three decades, in the kind of spacious house we had always dreamed of owning, life has been pretty good. I have been quite fortunate to have a loving, caring and supportive wife and children who bolstered me when the obsessions and compulsions became overwhelming. Despite all this, my troubles hardly went away with aging or changing careers.

In the spring of 2005, starting in my new career, my son and I traveled to Colorado's eastern edge to Holyoke, CO, at the behest of a good friend and golf course superintendent. He had accepted a job building a new course and wanted Jimmy and me to assist him. I was on hiatus from my regular monthly sessions with Dr. Lyons, because I had not been making any significant progress lately against OCD, and I was experiencing 25-35 incidents per day. The only activity that seemed to help was performing physical labor during twelve-hour days, leaving me with less time and physical or emotional energy for OCD interruptions. When the job building the golf course ended, I decided to complete a two-year online degree course from the University of Georgia, specializing in Golf Course Management. As I searched for work closer to home, my OCD came back forcefully. Not seeing Dr. Lyons on a regular basis turned out to have been a bad decision, because at least he could check to see if my medication was helping or needed to be adjusted. I began seeing Dr. Lyons regularly once again.

My dream of becoming an assistant golf course superintendent has not come to fruition, but I have been content working outdoors in an environment where no one bothers me. The peace and solitude of golf courses are much appreciated, along with enjoying the beauty of the landscape and surrounding nature. For five summers, I was privileged to work for my son, who had become an assistant superintendent, and I thoroughly enjoyed seeing him mature in his knowledge of the profession. A female employee once said to me, "Your son is the first superintendent I've worked with who takes the time to explain my job, so that I completely understand what I'm supposed to do. Jim is a great superintendent."

By 2008, Jimmy and I had helped build a second new golf course in Waterton Canyon, CO, a premiere foothills setting, with red rock formations rising throughout the course. Native spruce trees and grasses, along with pine trees, abound. The vistas, 30 miles from Denver, are breathtaking and the course is home to fox, deer, bighorn sheep, coyotes and the occasional bear, puma and rattlesnake.

Working on golf courses, I have had the opportunity to mentor many young co-workers, often college students, and have also befriended many in the golf maintenance industry who are alcoholics, past addicts or are individuals who have been in trouble with the law. During my lifetime, I have been employed in at least 40-50 occupations, from cleaning toilets to driving a trash truck to waiting tables and washing dishes. I have always been able to adapt successfully to the job, a chameleon in any situation. And yet, the harder I strived to be a better person, the worse the OCD symptoms became. In many ways, OCD is like alcoholism, drug addiction, severe illness or criminality. It changes a person's entire personality and never for the better. Perhaps I relate well to others who have suffered from these problems because of what I have lived through myself. My life experiences have given me empathy for people's struggles and pain and the challenges that always lie ahead.

On my 60th birthday, I was diagnosed with prostate cancer, but my primary physician thought it was treatable. When he informed me of the situation, I said, "Well, hell. That's quite a birthday surprise. Do you have any other secrets to tell me?"

After I received this diagnosis, for the first time in my life since childhood, the OCD obsessions and compulsions took a back seat. They didn't disappear, but diminished, which made me wonder if the only genuine 100% cure for OCD is death. At the same time, I felt confident that I wasn't going to die from cancer, but having cancer inevitably evoked many thoughts of my mortality. And Betsy and I were facing another problem. Prior to the diagnosis, I had applied for comprehensive medical coverage, which had a waiting period of several months. My medical coverage would cost $1,200 per month and—added to our other growing medical expenses—would leave us at least $75,000 in debt. The shock of not having insurance also pushed the OCD symptoms to the back of my mind.

In the times I have been most occupied during my life, mentally or physically or both, as when Betsy was preparing to give birth or when working at the golf course when my mother passed away, my OCD symptoms often, but not always, lessened in number and severity. What causes this particular phenomenon? When my brain is highly stimulated with a job or concentrating on something I enjoy, like coaching football, my mind is working so hard that the serotonin dysfunction is minimized. The OCD symptoms never disappear completely, but I am able to dismiss them more readily.

"When you get busy," Betsy has told me, "you don't have time to deal with the obsessions or compulsions. Time and again, I have seen this happen during our marriage."

God has always taken care of us financially, despite my never making much more than $50,000 a year while teaching and coaching. In 2009, facing down massive medical expenses, two very dear friends who were a married couple, came to our rescue. The wife worked for a well-known and highly-respected cancer specialist in Philadelphia who agreed to take me on as a pro bono patient. This physician ordered a full body scan for me to determine if the cancer had spread to any other organs, but the tests were negative. The doctor arranged for me to see another cancer specialist within his group to discuss several techniques for surgery and treatment. The specialist knew a cancer physician from Denver who was a pioneer in cryotherapy. I later reached out to the Denver specialist, since this procedure was less invasive than prostate removal surgery and produced excellent results. All the treatment in Philly was free of charge.

In the summer of 2009, I completed a two-year stint at a golf course quite far from home. After securing a raise and a job much nearer to my address, I am still employed there a decade later—the longest stretch I have ever worked anywhere. In the spring of 2010, I underwent cryotherapy cancer surgery and with the grace of God, a wonderful family, and dear friends I have been cancer-free for the past eight years. My OCD obsessions and compulsions, if lessened, were still present during this period of recovery, along with other challenging new realities. Prostate surgery was the beginning of the end of my sex life, as is often the norm.

Did this concern for my sexuality influence my OCD?

Yes.

Sex and the idea of committing mortal sins, attending confession and thoughts of sex with other women than my wife—all the usual symptoms came back with a vengeance in the next several years. I became the OCD poster boy for scrupulosity, forbidden thoughts and urges, and needing to talk about my past, present and future. With OCD a person does well for a while, partially controlling the obsessions, compulsions, rituals and all the other distractions. Then, like a wounded animal, OCD strikes with a ferocity that takes all the pleasures out of being alive, of being healthy, of being in love, of being successful, of being anything positive or good. OCD is an extension of evil. Do I really believe that? In part, I do.

By my mid-60's, I seriously doubted that I would ever have more control over my life. I had been disappointed on too many occasions, after having seen so many doctors and tried so many meds, which helped somewhat, but did not have lasting influences on my daily symptoms. My secret life was still winning the battle and my personal dreams of living a happy, exciting life without OCD were fading. I was running out of time, and my eternal optimism was departing.

I sensed that Betsy had also become tired and overwhelmed by my depressed and fractious behavior. We both wondered if this was all life had to offer in our "Golden Years?" Optimism was all but gone.

A religious adage I recall states something like, "God never allows a person to face a burden unless he/she possesses the strength and wherewithal to carry that burden and live productively while dealing with it."

I believe those words, but God had definitely tested Betsy and me to our limits. My personal strength and perseverance to cope originally came from my parents. Then it came from Betsy, who had unconditionally loved and supported me every day of my life since we had met. Then it came from our four loving, empathetic children and a plethora of devoted family and friends. I would not be alive without these individuals and cannot fathom how those without such loving support can live with OCD. One of the most effective sources of love and compassion the past thirteen years has been our three grandchildren: thirteen, twelve, and nine. Without being overly involved or spoiling them, Betsy and I are as dedicated and devoted to their happiness and well-being as possible. Our grandchildren's love and presence has strengthened my determination to control and overcome my OCD.

By the end of 2011, the prostate cancer was gone. I was seeing my psychiatrist, Dr. Lyons, about once a month and had continued daily on Lexapro, which helped calm me in situations that might have become confrontational. The superintendent of the course where I worked for four summers had a very volatile personality, especially with those on the grounds crew. The truth is that I saw much of myself in him when I was in my early forties because he had a propensity to lose his temper and shout when everyday mistakes were made; overreacting to problems that did not warrant this level of anger. I saw several good employees quit their jobs.

For the first couple of years of his tenure, I was the recipient of his wrath, as he occasionally reprimanded me, threatened to fire me, and challenged my fitness for the job. Not once in the eleven years to date, of my employment under this man, have I raised my voice or responded to him with any aggression. One summer, a few weeks after overreacting and reprimanding me, he said to me, "Coach, I don't know how you can stand the criticism the way you do. If I were you, I would have quit." He smiled and drove off in his golf cart, leaving me bewildered, but thankful for my calmness with him.

More than once, I have asked myself why I put up with his behavior. Well, I like my job, it is close to home, and I make decent money. I collect unemployment in the off-season; I am not really harmed by his criticism, and have wanted to prove to myself that I can remain in one place of employment for more than a few years. And low and behold my supervisor saw the error of his ways, and has become an exemplary boss and exceptional leader. And we are now friends who respect one another.

During these fifteen years, our youngest daughter graduated with a degree in education after working almost full-time and attending school for seven years. She teaches elementary school with and has befriended one of my former high school pupils. Once or twice a year, she invites me to visit her classroom to teach a history class. Our only son, Jimmy, explored in Thailand, Cambodia and Vietnam one summer, visiting shrines and the infamous Hanoi Hilton Prison, where Senator John McCain was held for years during the Vietnam War. During another summer, Jimmy secured a job teaching at an English language school in Costa Rica and worked in a turtle conservatory, before graduating from Metropolitan State University in Denver, magna cum laude. Around this time, our third grandchild was born.

From 2011 through 2014, my OCD wasn't gone, but was not always overwhelming. Yet at times, it was. While watching television, I would watch a scene triggering sexual thoughts or obsessions. I would tell my mind that I did not want to commit a sin, or had not already committed a mortal sin by viewing two scantily-clad individuals making love. When I could not dismiss the obsession immediately, the compulsions began in earnest. I would have had to get up and leave the family room, walk to the bathroom, close the door, stare at the wall and convince myself that I hadn't sinned. Sometimes, it took several minutes to push the compulsion out of my thinking, before I could return to the show.

My obsessions almost always involved women, sex and mortal sin. Incidents like this were starting to number 30-40 a day, or even more, despite my growing older and taking a sizable dose of Lexapro every evening. I kept asking myself, just as I had been doing for decades: when am I going to find relief from my obsessions and compulsions? When are the OCD rituals ever going to end? I have a loving wife, four beautiful children, and three precious grandchildren. I want to enjoy my life and the last couple of decades on earth, and have much that I still want to accomplish. Can anything—or anyone—help me?

To say I was becoming more and more despondent doesn't fully convey my mindset. I was flat-out desperate to end my secret life!

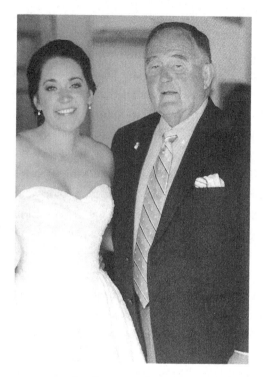

Stephanie and Author
Lake Granby, CO, June 20, 2015

Chapter XIII

# Bottom of the Barrel

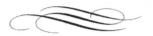

*B*etween the year I was found to be free of prostate cancer and the beginning of 2015, I had several aged-related maladies and surgeries. In early 2013, I was scheduled to have a small metal plate affixed to three neck vertebrae to alleviate nerve problems in my arm and hand. The morning prior to the neck surgery, I awoke deathly nauseous and dizzy, without hearing in one ear. A virus had attacked this ear and despite a steroid shot and numerous tests, my hearing was gone and I had to begin to wear hearing aids. The hearing in my other ear is 75-80%.

Following successful neck surgery, I had a rotator cuff operation on one shoulder and a less invasive bone procedure on the other. After years of random bouts of dizziness and light-headedness, and having to wear a heart monitor while working, I was diagnosed with atrial fibrillation, now controlled with medication. Lastly, I suffer from sleep apnea —a serious deficit of oxygen to the internal organs while asleep. I utilize a CPAP machine which supplies sufficient oxygen as I sleep. All of these ailments pale in comparison to living with OCD.

In April of 2015, I was invited to be part of a three-day reunion of my high school classmates at one of their homes in the Ojai Valley of California, just east of the Pacific Ocean and Santa Barbara, CA. Eight guys in their late sixties came together to plan our 50th high school reunion, commemorating graduation from an all-male college prep school in the Washington D.C. suburbs, Georgetown Preparatory School. Each of us met with at least two or three classmates we had not seen or talked with in 48 years—our days filled with talking, laughing, joking and shedding a few tears over accomplishments and disappointments. We toured the rolling hills surrounding Ojai, bordered by acre after acre of citrus trees, avocado orchards, and wine vineyards, visiting the renowned coastal town of Santa Barbara and eating fresh seafood in a restaurant on the Pacific shore. Several of the men were my closest high school friends and the emotions of our get-together bolstered me for my coming showdown with OCD.

I returned home to Denver and Betsy and I made plans for our youngest daughter's wedding in June at a lakeside mountain resort. The bridegroom was a life-long family friend—caring, kind and hard-working. When I should have felt joyful over these developments, I was overwhelmed by the frequency and severity of OCD incidents—depressed, anxious, angry, frustrated, sullen and preoccupied, with occasional thoughts of suicide.

At this age, women still continued to make me nervous and uncomfortable. The more attractive the woman, the more uncomfortable I became. Like clock-work, whenever I went out to dinner, I experienced an attraction to one or more of the prettier waitresses and thought about dating or running away with one of them. This has been part of my dining experience for at least the past 50 years. How can I be 70 and still fantasize about running off with the cute 30-year-old at the local pub? This habit has saddled me with guilt since I was a teenager.

Why in the hell," I repeatedly inquire of myself, "can't I just eat in peace?"

Several months prior to the wedding, Betsy, myself, our daughter and future son-in-law, Gregory, visited the beautiful mountain town of Grand Lake, the site of the wedding and one of Colorado's most scenic spots. The lake is reputed to be the deepest lake in the state, surrounded on three sides by majestic snow-covered, 14,000-foot Rocky Mountain peaks. The wedding church was a block from the lake shore and the venue for the reception provided spectacular views of the mountains reflected on the surface of the lake.

The wedding priest was tall and handsome, in his late forties, with Catholic values on the sanctity and importance of marriage. He held traditional church beliefs on all seven sacraments, including the Sacrament of Confession, entangled within me since childhood. I had probably made my last confession a year or two before. Prior to meeting this priest, my OCD incidents had been steadily rising to 50-70 per day, with repetitive obsessions, compulsions and rituals involving sexual thoughts, mortal sins and returning to confession to save my soul from hell.

I was obsessed with confessing my sins and asking for forgiveness in the Sacrament of Penance. As I matured through the years, I had grown more and more ashamed of my actions and more and more embarrassed to tell them to a priest in a confessional, especially those related to sex. I would have been much more comfortable confessing to grand larceny or murder. Leading up to the wedding, I went to church and made what I hoped was a good, honest confession, stating that I suffered from OCD. The priest seemed understanding, expressing compassion and forgiving me for my sins. I had said my Act of Contrition Prayer, but still believed this wasn't sufficient because I had not told the priest the whole truth, or given enough detail, about my sins regarding sex. Following this, I had multiple incidents and obsessions/compulsions/thoughts about not making an honest and good confession. They increased as the wedding approached.

The week of the nuptials, I took off Thursday through Monday from work at the golf course. Sixteen of our family members met in Grand Lake at a three-story home, a cool breeze rippling off the lake and into the house. I affixed an Italian flag horizontally along the outside railing of the porch, so family and visitors would recognize the wedding headquarters. Relatives arrived all the way from southern New Jersey, along with 120 other guests. A deep feeling of peace and contentment began to surround me finally.

Friday began with a magnificent sunrise over the mountain peaks, rising and exploding over the continental divide and falling on the glass-like stillness of the lake. The scent of spruce and pine permeated the air. My uncle Charles, always the most mellow and compassionate of the six siblings in my father's family, had helped me navigate my often turbulent relationship with my dad. Charles too had symptoms of OCD and I had always loved and admired Charles for his empathy and caring personality. He was a hugger, and "I love you" type of man, and my go-to friend. Seeing him should have made me happy, but there were complications.

Over the years during social gatherings—holiday parties, family gatherings or celebrations—my OCD and obsessions/compulsions would quite often become more intense and numerous. My daughter's nuptials became a constant, ongoing tug-of-war between unwanted, constant and repetitive obsessions about sex, which led to unwanted, constant and repetitive compulsions or rituals to rid myself of such thoughts. The "master" of hiding or disguising OCD symptoms was put to the ultimate test to cover up the negative obsessions and compulsions raging in his head, while attempting to show enjoyment and love for many, many special moments and people. What a complete and utter waste, an abomination. The wedding turned into my personal conflict of good versus evil inside my own mind.

I also recall seeing my daughter, radiant and perfectly beautiful in her wedding dress. I remember my own timid efforts to mollify her nervousness while walking down the church aisle, so proud of her. I had choked up at the podium saying prayers for departed family members, especially my mother and father, and I remember how amazed I was when our five-year-old grandson responded to a request from the priest for prayers for the couple and said, "I hope Aunt Stephie and Uncle Greggy have a very happy life together."

I recollect the first father/daughter dance with the bride to our favorite Paul Simon song and the same grandson break dancing for over two hours, before asking permission to lie down. Yet throughout the event the OCD was winning.

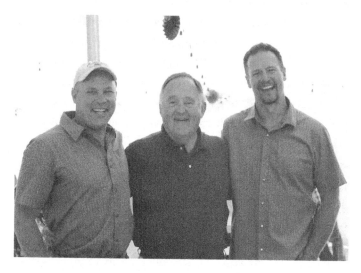

L-R: Greg Shaw, Author, Rob Neiberger
Granby, CO, June 2018

## Chapter XIV

# Hope... At Last

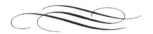

*B*y mid-2015, I had been seeing and receiving superb counseling and medication for OCD from the same psychiatrist for nineteen years. Doctor Lyons had prescribed Lexapro, which I had been taking for the past five years. But now the OCD incidents had increased to where I was desperate and overwhelmed by their frequency and severity. I was obsessed with simply attempting to make it through each day, with more thoughts of suicide. Following my daughter's wedding, my symptoms spun out of control and I saw Doctor Lyons, who steered me toward an expert in OCD therapy, Dr. Gallagher, the region's foremost expert in ERP, Exposure Response Prevention Therapy. Dr. Lyons explained to Betsy and me that Dr. Gallagher's therapy was somewhat unconventional, but he, Dr. Lyons, thought I might be finally ready to investigate Dr. Gallagher's techniques. Dr. Lyons also asked me to try a new anti-depressant, Cymbalta, and that July I began taking 60 mgs of Cymbalta, once a day, which I continue to use.

In August, Betsy and I met initially with Dr. Gallagher for an hour. He was frank in explaining his ground rules: he would be asking me to take actions no one ever had. He expected

tion and if I would meet his requirements,
ntee that he could help me. Within the first few
our initial meeting, I knew that I liked him and
could work with him. He described my condition this way;
"OCD is a phobia which lives in a place in a person where
that person is least open and most vulnerable. It can only exist
if the host individual displays these three characteristics to
OCD: resistance, avoidance and escape, the three fuels which
feed the engine of OCD."

My wife sat dumbfounded in Dr. Gallagher's office, not
believing for a moment that I would agree to his demands.
Dr. Lyons and Betsy thought my strong Catholic upbringing
would prevent me from doing what Dr. Gallagher was
suggesting, but I had kept, even from them just how much
my secret life tormented me. I was ready for any therapy if it
could minimize or eliminate my symptoms.

I told Dr. Gallagher, "I am at a point in my life where I will
try just about anything to beat my OCD. I will do whatever
you say, if it will help me get rid of it."

From Dr. Jim Gallagher:

*I was born in 1967 on Long Island and attended New York's
Oneonta State College before earning my graduate degree from
the University of Denver's School of Professional Psychology.
While doing research in Boston at the National Center for
Post-Traumatic Stress Disorder, I realized that my true passion
was clinical work. I returned to Colorado to start a private prac-
tice and have had my own Denver office for the past 23 years.
I specialize in the behavioral treatment of anxiety disorders;*

*specifically, exposure-based interventions. Of the thousands of psychologists or psychiatrists in the metropolitan area, I'm one of only a handful doing Exposure with Response Prevention (ERP). Despite being the most empirically supported treatment for anxiety disorders, much of the therapeutic community still considers ERP to be too taxing on the patient, and, I would also say, on the average clinician. It can be difficult work and is still considered radical in some camps. It is "radical" in the true meaning of the word, as it gets to "the root" of the factors that maintain anxiety disorders. Most clinicians are trained to think that anxiety is the problem to be managed and contained. Anxiety is never the problem. The culturally-sanctioned agenda to avoid anxiety-evoking stimuli is the problem. As such, I am an anxiety disorder specialist who doesn't believe in "anxiety disorders." I treat anxiety avoidance disorders.*

*I came to ERP in 1991 in graduate school, drawn to it because of its effectiveness. ERP for the treatment of Obsessive Compulsive Disorder is on average 85% effective in remitting 80% of OCD symptomatology. In contrast, while medication can often serve as a helpful adjunct, it has only a 50% chance of working at all and a best outcome is usually a 35% reduction in symptoms. No treatment on the psychological market comes close to ERP. It is fundamentally based upon the premise that if you truly embrace and face the thing you're most afraid of, you'll change your relationship with it and its capacity to engender more fear responses. What one resists, persists...be it a thought, an emotion or a physical sensation. OCD-type thoughts have actually been empirically demonstrated to be common in non-clinical populations. What distinguishes OCD sufferers is the level to which they try to avoid and escape their unwanted thoughts and emotions.*

*Many clinicians and clients have a culturally reinforced resistance to ERP because it can be very uncomfortable. As such, I encourage people to go outside the cultural norm. From this perspective, ERP is not "normal" in the literal sense of the word. However, there is a concept within psychology gaining increasing support known as "destructive normality," meaning that some "normal" psychological and behavioral strategies for managing thoughts and emotions can cause needless suffering. Escape and avoidance are the top contenders.*

*So yes, I have been known to expose people with contamination fears of public toilets to confront this by licking them. I have exposed countless loving mothers tortured by unwanted thoughts of murdering their children to explicit and detailed audiotaped scripts of potentially doing the act itself. I get in the car with people who've had vehicular accidents and walk them through the wreck and all the possible worst-case scenarios. I expose survivors of sexual assault to imaginatively reliving the event a hundred times. I treat individuals afraid of passing out by having them intentionally hyperventilate in public. I deliberately induce panic symptoms in those afraid of panic attacks. I have people who suffer from social anxiety recite poetry at the top of their lungs or call out the time of day every minute on the minute in Target and Home Depot. I show them, on a fundamental, visceral level, that other people's negative evaluations do not matter. And in so doing, they become free of further suffering in this regard.*

On our second visit to Dr. Gallagher, he said we were going

"on a field trip." The three of us immediately got in our car and he directed us to the nearest Barnes and Noble Bookstore. Leaving Betsy in the car, I followed him inside and he led me to "men's magazines." He picked out three different editions of *Playboy* and we began to view the contents. After several minutes, he said, "What do you think? Should we buy them?"

"Sure," I replied, confused and somewhat at a loss for words.

He took the magazines to the cashier, paid for them, and we went back to his office. Betsy remained in the car and he gave me homework prior to our next scheduled visit: read the magazine articles and view and enjoy all the photographs. He also presented me with the addresses of the most popular and most watched pornographic websites. This was the start of my personal course in "exposure and response prevention therapy."

From Dr. Jim Gallagher:

*Jim came to me as a lifelong coach of young men so I mirrored that back to him by becoming his ERP coach. His basic problem was that he was compulsively avoiding and/or escaping any sexually-related thought or experience that would potentially result in damning his immortal soul to hell. As is the case with many OCD sufferers, he displayed a cognitive pattern of "thought-action fusion"—he believed that thinking something was equivalent to doing the act itself. What distinguished Jim from nearly all OCD patients was his capacity for aggression. The vast majority of OCD sufferers are passive* and shy, and often Good Samaritans. The last thing they want is to harm another person. Jim is very rare because he suffers from both OCD and anger management issues. In 23 years of treating OCD patients, I've only seen three people with this combination, so that made him more challenging.

Jim is a really tough human being, in the true sense of the word, and his toughness and sheer tenacity have kept him alive when a lot of people would have committed suicide. He lived and suffered with this for many decades, despite having actively sought treatment. Jim has clearly demonstrated that after so much suffering, one can find adequate care and recover. His recovery has been remarkable to witness and I feel very privileged and honored by being part of his process.

The first time he and Betsy came to my office, she was very quiet, barely talking at all. Jim presented as not having any knowledge of ERP—he knew nothing about the kind of work I do so he had no preconceptions. He demonstrated a fairly high level of "overvalued ideation," in which the individual lacks the awareness of the potential absurdity of his thoughts and feelings.

During our initial session, I used a coaching model as a metaphor for treatment. I suggested that the best coaches push players to their perceived limit and then a little bit beyond, but not to the point where they would want to quit. I challenged him hard, much harder than I normally would. I tried to harness his toughness and ability to fight, viewing them as strengths versus liabilities in his treatment. I challenged him as a man. I said you have to ball up—no complaining or whining. I said that if he did exactly what I told him to do we weren't going to injure his OCD we were going to kill it. And, *most importantly, we were going to operate as if there's no hell. I flooded him with his most feared thoughts. You sinned...A Lot. I would often say, "Jim, you're really fucked now. You're so fucked, so fucked." I also helped him develop a more workable relationship with God.*

*I told him that if God is the most all-powerful and totally efficient force in the universe, then he has got to have the best game in town. At the very least, God has to have a better game than I do. From a learning and theoretical level, it has been well established in empirical literature that punishment is the weakest method of modifying human behavior. But if you are going to use it, it is critical to apply it at maximal intensity during the time closet to the undesired behavior. So to punish someone for having a sexual thought decades ago by sending him to hell 60 or 70 years later made Jim's view of God... well, I would say...completely moronic. Presented this way, Jim understood what I was saying.*

*As a method of systematically exposing Jim to unwanted sexual thoughts and extinguishing his avoidance behavior around this stimuli, I had him look at pornographic magazines in increasingly more public places—first at Barnes and Noble and then at Starbuck's. We progressed to him watching pornographic videos. I also did audio, talking with Jim about going to hell for doing these things and showing him how language can be de-literalized. My purpose was this: if I can trigger the fear inside of someone, I can treat it, so that's what I did with him.*

*On a very basic level, inside the human brain the amygdala sends signals to the hippocampus about what is emotion-*

*ally important or not important. Each pathway has its own distinct "library" of stored information as to why that may or may not be the case. Non-reinforced exposure to fear-provoking stimuli (exposure to a stimulus that is a false predictor of harm in the absence of harm) essentially retrains the brain on this most fundamental level. In other words, we train the amygdala to recognize that a stimulus, one is exposed to, is no longer a predictor of harm. For example, if you've been beaten by a baseball bat, I expose you to a bat and show you that it's not dangerous now, so it's no longer a predictor of harm.*

*OCD lives in that place where one is not experientially willing to go. It feeds off all the thoughts and feelings a person is unwilling to experience, and as such, the brain deems them dangerous. I expose patients to all the private events that are resisted and people learn that they are not predictors of danger or harm. This awareness or understanding may occur at any age, regardless of the length of time from the original onset of OCD. From this perspective, psychological health is defined as being able to think and feel anything, anywhere, at any intensity and for any duration—with no defense.*

Until now, I had never purchased a *Playboy*, been on a pornographic website or watched porn in any form. I had looked at a *Playboy* perhaps six or eight times, but now I was engaging in activities totally foreign to me and in violation of the rules and regulations of Catholicism. Dr. Gallagher had placed a forbidden order for me on all praying, attending church, and, most especially, attending confession. I was being forced to abandon many of my most precious and important personal habits. Obeying these dictates wasn't easy and my actions were not free of severe doubt and guilt. But I trusted him and did what he said, perusing the magazines often, always in secret, and regularly viewing pornography via the internet, again always in secret. What I saw on these websites was beyond my wildest imaginings. I now joke with my wife that, "I watch porn to keep my OCD in check."

Let me be very clear, I consider pornography vile, immoral and personally repugnant. For someone who once considered himself a very devout Catholic—close to God and his religion—to be forced to rely upon viewing such things to keep his brain chemicals in balance is both ironic and abhorrent. I despise what I have to look at, but do it out of necessity and a genuine desire to live a more enjoyable and productive life. I'm sacrificing a small piece of myself as a decent person to be a more loving and caring husband, father, grandfather and friend. I'm making up for the thousands of memorable moments lost in my life due to OCD symptoms and transgressions. I will suffer any consequences in front of me to improve the time left with my family.

For all practical purposes, my OCD has remained in check with just a few instances of obsessions and compulsions. I sometimes say to myself, "Is this life I'm now living, really and truly my life?" The answer, unequivocally, is yes. Where was Dr. Gallagher and exposure response prevention therapy for the last 55 years?

When watching pornography, I am purposely exposing my brain to fear-provoking situations, which appears to teach my brain's circuitry to unlearn the dysfunctional behaviors of obsessions and compulsions. Exposure and response prevention therapy enhances emotional or positive learning by altering faulty connections in these circuits. Anti-depressant and anti-psychotic medications also target the activity of regulating neurotransmitters, so my brain will not force unwanted obsessions or compulsions upon me.

After taking Cymbalta while participating in ERP for less than a year, my OCD incidents began to diminish—almost immediately. In the beginning, I saw Doctor Gallagher once a week, for 50 minutes, for several months. Then, after improving significantly, I began seeing him only once a month for the past three years. At present we meet and talk every five weeks or so. I have progressed from having an average of 60 to 65 OCD incidents per day, to an average of 1-2 incidents. I am happier today than at any time since grade school. I have my life back, and I am mentally and physically free to devote myself to my family, friends and those daily activities which were constantly interrupted and often destroyed.

My wife and our four adult children will tell you I am a changed man. Life-long close friends and relatives, teaching and coaching colleagues and more recent acquaintances, do not see a significant change in my demeanor, because for most of my life, I was excellent in disguising my OCD. My entire public life and career were built around cleverly hidden secrets. I became an expert in deception because time after time when I have finally disclosed to my closest life-long friends that I have suffered from OCD all of my life, they say, "I never knew you had that. I had no clue."

From Betsy:

When Dr. Lyons changed Jim's medication and then suggested he meet with Dr. Gallagher, neither one of us had any idea what we were in for. Dr. Lyons had told us that it might take awhile to see Dr. Gallagher, as he was very busy, as long as six to twelve months.

I called the next day and left a message with Dr. Gallagher, giving him some specifics about Jim and his OCD symptoms. Unbelievably, he called the very next day and set up an appointment for us the following week. We were both shocked, but later found out that Dr. Gallagher took us so quickly because of Jim's age, how long he'd been suffering with OCD, and because Dr. Gallagher was convinced he could help him.

Both of us went to the first meeting and I remember saying to Jim, "Are you sure you're going to be able to do all of this? Are you sure you want to do this?"

I knew Jim well enough to know that what Dr. Gallagher was asking of him, was the furthest thing from my mind. When Dr. Gallagher asked me what I thought my response was, "I just want this to go away!"

Jim said something else: he was beyond done with everything else and would try anything now.

It's amazing to me how fast—using Dr. Gallagher's therapy—Jim's OCD disappeared. He's almost entirely free of his symptoms and has become the person I always knew he was. It's also amazing how well he disguised his OCD for all those years. If you asked his football players and/or students, they'll tell you he was the best coach/teacher they ever had, and his friends will say the same thing. Jim is finally able to see what everyone else sees in him—even if it was hidden from him for *so long. I only hope he can live the rest of his life OCD free.*

*So here we are, 55 years after meeting and we both can honestly say that he's found peace of mind. He is that warm, fun, loving and caring guy I met all those decades ago, but now he's so much more and able to live the life he should have been living all along. He doesn't get angry at the smallest things and is always present when you're talking to him. He laughs so much more than before, trying to get as much joy out of life as he can.*

*All I can say is, "It was worth the wait!"*

I am much calmer and more at peace after seeing Dr. Gallagher. I am less stressed and rarely lose my patience and temper. I'm far quieter, more contemplative, less distracted, can make fun of myself and I'm more receptive to new acquaintances. Sometimes, I sleep too often, lack energy or binge eat sweets and I'm easily bored, at times, but none of the symptoms approach what I used to have on a daily basis.

At age 66 ½, I finally met a doctor who was an expert in the treatment of OCD. Finding Dr. Gallagher and being willing to try ERP Therapy has provided for my family and me an entirely new life, almost totally devoid of a horrible curse.

After practicing the ERP Therapy for a year, I went to my eye doctor's office and was seen by an attractive female nurse's aide. While I was in the examination room with my wife, the aide placed a tissue in my left hand, after administering eye drops, an act of simple courtesy for a patient with tears in his eyes. I experienced an OCD incident, but for less than 30 seconds. My ERP training allowed me to say to myself, "You did not commit a moral sin by allowing the nurse's aide to touch your hand and possibly your thigh when she placed the Kleenex into your hand and if you did commit a mortal sin, so what? No big deal. You are not going to hell because her hand may have possibly touched you."

Hope most definitely exists for people suffering from OCD!

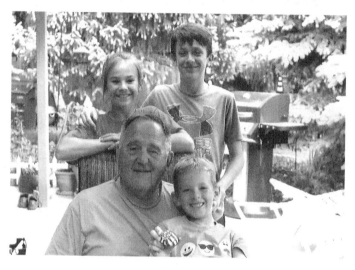

L-R: Stella, Cooper, Author, Trevor
Littleton, CO, 2018

## Epilogue

# Counsel and Advice

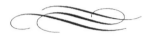

What do the next years have in store for me? I am not psychic, but now I possess some of the intricate formula that has unlocked my life's greatest mystery. I will continue to follow to the letter the precepts of ERP as prescribed by Dr. Gallagher and to take the medication enabling me to lessen many of my OCD symptoms.

A long time ago, I created a written pledge for the athletes I coached, which they'd recite before every practice and each game. Several high school head coaches borrowed it for their squads and this pledge may be applicable for certain OCD sufferers:

### SUCCESS PLEDGE

*"I am a good person. I will always display courage and strength in my life's endeavors. I will show determination at all times. I will have confidence in myself, in my family and in my doctors. I am a winner. I will always act like a winner both at home and in public. I will <u>never</u> give up. I will forever strive to overcome OCD. I possess the main ingredient of a champion, PRIDE. I am a champion! I will triumph over OCD."*

This mantra should be recited whenever OCD symptoms or its influence seems to be overwhelming an individual with OCD.

Dr. Gallagher has often told me that OCD treatment is not easy.

"ERP therapy," he says, "is like trying to hold patients' heads under water all day."

He's described one group of OCD patients as meek, fearful and unable to confront their most serious problems. Some of them suffer from mental illnesses or phobias, but refuse to seek professional help. He calls them "recovery avoiders" or RA's. The two most important aspects of OCD which need to be understood today by all individuals are:

1. THE DEGREE OF PAIN AND SUFFERING OCD CAUSES PATIENTS IS IMMEASURABLE; OCD IS INSIDIOUS AND UNRELENTING.

2. THE COMPLEXITY OF OCD AND THE PERSONAL SECRECY IT CREATES WITHIN PATIENTS REQUIRES MUCH LOVE, PATIENCE AND CONSTANT WORK AS WELL AS PERSEVERANCE BY SUFFERERS AND THEIR LOVED ONES IN ORDER TO OVERCOME THE OCD.

The vast majority of American citizens, including spouses and parents, have no clue regarding OCD, its symptoms, and its negative effects on sufferers. Even well-educated individuals know very little about its life-changing debilitation. Most OCD patients suffer in silence and many of them are mild and gentle people. OCD seems to prey on the meek and submissive. Dr. Gallagher has confided in me that in his twenty-three years of dealing with OCD patients, he has only worked with a very few like me, who are tough and determined to control their OCD, rather than the other way around. Recent mental health studies for the U.S. indicate there are three million OCD sufferers, ages 18-54. My personal estimate, because so many live secret lives, would double that figure. OCD patients are ten times more likely to commit suicide than other mental health patients. And 90% of all suicides in the United States today include individuals who suffer from some type of mental disorder, which includes OCD.

Dr. Gallagher has told Betsy and me that over my lifetime, I have been a prime candidate for suicide. I believe my faith in God and an ongoing belief in my overcoming OCD prevented me from killing myself, along with Betsy's love and devotion, which have been my defining source of courage. Without her, I would not be here.

My heartfelt advice to OCD sufferers is this: Never permit yourself to be passive when dealing with this condition. Take your frustration, anger, despair or any other negative emotion you may be experiencing and find someone—a family member, close friend, colleague or soul mate—and confide in him/her honestly. This can be difficult to follow, but can be the initial step in helping yourself become well. Remind yourself that you are not a bad person because you have OCD or because your brain chemicals are deficient. Acknowledge that your OCD is not due to anything you have ever done, but the result of a brain dysfunction, just as some people are born left-handed or require glasses. Do not give in to denial, but face OCD head-on.

After admitting you have a problem, you should talk to someone you trust about your most intimate secrets. Then find the courage, with the assistance of the listener, to seek professional help and guidance. Do not feel embarrassed or intimidated by this process. Thousands of health professionals are willing to help with OCD—offering a multitude of therapies and approaches to deal successfully with its many variations. Dr. Gallagher has told me that SRI's taken to reduce OCD symptoms are only about 35% effective. If one med doesn't work, try another. New and more effective medications are now available. Also, find the doctor who most effectively meets your needs. This has to be someone with whom you feel comfortable and in whom you have the most confidence. I have been treated by seven different doctors throughout my struggles with OCD. Betsy and I never developed a sincere relationship with our doctor under the guidance of several of them. I did not meet Dr. Lyons until I was nearly fifty, and he didn't think that I was ready to work with Dr. Gallagher and ERP Therapy until my mid-sixties.

Please understand that I am an OCD individual and OCD sufferer. I do not use the term "patient" because for me, that word denotes there is something inherently wrong with me. While I understand that I have a disorder, I have always tried to live my life as a moral and somewhat normal human being. I may very well have inherited OCD from my father or his family, long before it was understood, and most certainly before doctors and medical researchers had any clue about what caused it.

Do I suffer from a mental illness? Yes, I do. However, throughout my secret life with OCD, I have refrained from admitting that I have a form of mental illness, because I had no intention of giving into that notion. Yet I readily acknowledge that I have a chemical abnormality within my brain, which directly and indirectly affects my behavior. This disorder or mental health phobia caused my obsessions and ritualistic compulsions.

Do I think of myself as disabled because of obsessive compulsive disorder? My OCD has never totally disabled me, but for many people, OCD must be viewed as a disability. A person who cannot hold a job and make a living, or who is a recluse trapped inside his home due to OCD, must be considered disabled. These people too have a secret life—and living that secret life is one of the many common symptoms of OCD, much like anxiety, depression and anger.

No psychiatrist, no psychologist, no parent or family member, no human being who doesn't suffer from OCD, can realistically understand the insidiousness, the intensity or level of debilitation the disorder brings. Doctors, clinicians, relatives, and friends can try, but they can never grasp the repercussions of losing a limb unless they have lost one. Hundreds of times throughout my mysterious journey—as a child, adolescent, young adult and mature adult—I have gone down on my knees and begged God to take this affliction from me. If brain surgery allowed doctors to remove the part of me that causes OCD, I would have signed up for the surgery long ago!

How many days have I sat across from a physician, a specialist, my wife or one of my children and looked them in the eye and admitted how utterly asinine my ritualistic obsessions and/or behaviors actually are? Yet I had little or no control in ending them once and for all. I hated that feeling of powerlessness and deeply resented this intrusion into my life.

In the summer of 2018, my younger brother David, who was mentally disabled, began to experience eating problems and had to be fed with a tube. More complications developed with recurring pneumonia, and as his legal guardian I was forced to confront the dilemma of whether or not his quality of life was ever going to improve. After consulting with my brother's two primary physicians, I concluded the answer was no. I decided, after considering many factors, that I would place him in hospice care and allow him to die peacefully and without pain. In my heart, I knew that my parents, who had left me to care for David, just as they had many times when he was an infant and I was an adolescent, would not have wanted him to suffer anymore.

I spent the next three weeks sitting with David every day. Although he had never spoken a word nor shown recognition for any family member, including my parents, I realized now that he knew my voice and that I was there with him. One day an orderly who'd been caring for him for years walked past his room and loudly called out, "Hey David, how are you, my man?" the orderly waved to David. The man stopped at the door and David looked right at him, raised his hand, and pointed as if giving a high-five. At that moment, I knew David recognized his friend.

Those three weeks I shared with my 60-year-old disabled little brother became a truly wonderful time. I came to realize just how special his life was and how fortunate I was to be enjoying myself without the daily OCD obsessions and compulsions. I was able to share the end of my brother's life in a peaceful fashion, while looking forward to sharing the remainder of mine with my wife, children and grandchildren. I realized how much I had accomplished by getting my OCD under control.

Every significant experience in a person's life, I believe happens for a reason. My battle with OCD had greatly improved over the preceding two-and-a-half years, so that I could fulfill my responsibility and promise to my parents and take care of David. He died peacefully in his sleep on July 16, 2018 and was laid to rest three days later with our parents and an infant sibling in a private gravesite ceremony. On his headstone below his name are the words, "A SAINT ON EARTH."

Whenever I sit and discuss a topic with our three grandchildren, I am rewarded by having refused to let OCD dominate my life. Private time with my wife is much more meaningful now and our love for one another is stronger than ever. I relish each opportunity to be with our children and their spouses.

The most important aspect of my life as a youngster was unquestionably my relationship with God and my Catholic faith. Serving mass was more important to me than playing football, which was my passion. Participating in church ceremonies as an altar boy made me feel more spiritual, as if I were functioning on a higher level. In adulthood, I experienced similar feelings as a theology teacher and acting as a communion minister. Yet over the decades my life as a faithful Catholic has disintegrated considerably. Peace of mind and escaping OCD have been achieved not through the religious rituals of my youth, but through watching pornography, of all things. This is not how I ever imagined my life unfolding— but life is what it is. Going forward, my goal is to love and enjoy my wife, children, grandchildren and friends as much as possible, using my health and good fortune to continue as a mentor, coach and caring individual.

How do I rectify being a man of faith and strong values with periodically viewing pornography in order to keep my OCD under control? I do so by believing that I remain an empathetic and compassionate person. The difference now is that I no longer must live a secret life. I do what is required to control the OCD symptoms and play catch-up with my real life.

Lastly, in my wallet today I carry an Organ Donor for Research Card and have arranged upon my death for my brain to be donated to the NIH Brain and Tissue Depository in California. I hope through the study of my brain, some answers may be found to help researchers determine how to more effectively understand and control OCD.

To all who have suffered pieces of what I have: Be strong, seek help and never give up the fight!

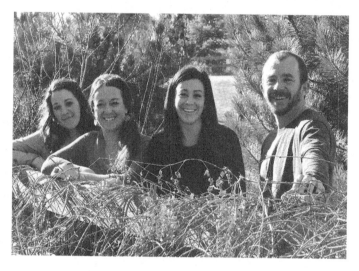

L-R: Stephanie, Amy, Laura, Jimmy
Ft. Collins, CO

# Testimonials
# from Jim and Betsy's Children

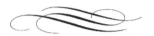

*F*rom Jim's Oldest Daughter Amy:

*I've had a very good life and was brought up by two amazing parents. Being the oldest of four siblings and helping around the house with the younger kids, I became acutely aware of what was going around me. Around seven or eight, I realized that Dad was battling something. I didn't know what it was, but always felt so badly for him and the need to help him. At times, he'd get really angry, punching holes in walls, hitting himself, and yelling at Mom or others in our family. I knew it wasn't anything we'd done, but something deeper which he couldn't control, something he was born with.*

*While getting my B.A. in Psychology at Denver University, I began learning more about OCD. I remember sitting in my dorm room and crying after reading a chapter on OCD and knowing what Dad had been through for decades, while raising a family and nurturing a teaching/coaching career. He was never anything but loving and protective of me, and in time I realized that he was my hero for dealing with and ulti-*

*mately overcoming the trials of this disease. I'm so thankful that he found Dr. Gallagher and for the help he's given Dad. My father seems like a new person and much happier now, with this insane amount of weight lifted from his shoulders.*

*Dad, I know what you've endured and I'm so proud of you. It takes a very strong person to confront and conquer what you've been through and I'm so glad you've finally found freedom from OCD. I hope this book can help others dealing with this illness. I love you Dad—you are the best!*

From Jim's Youngest Daughter Stephanie:

*Unfortunately, as kids I don't think we knew the severity of Dad's OCD. What he was doing just seemed normal to us. Growing up, we always joked about the obsessive things Dad did and also joked that we had this condition as well. Now as an adult, I'm noticing these obsessive traits coming out not only in myself, but in my siblings. As a teacher, I find it difficult to let go of work that needs to get done. It's a job that never ends, so in my mind there's this uncontrollable feeling of wanting to do more and more, resulting in an unhappy and unbalanced lifestyle. In order to control this, I have to create to-do lists putting things in terms of priority. I give myself only a certain amount of time each day to complete these tasks or I'd never stop. Once the time is up, I tell myself to walk away. It's not easy, and I don't always follow this routine because I want everything to be perfect and completing my work brings me satisfaction. I have to remind myself that my life and my time are just as important as the time I put into my students.*

*It's time I can't get back, so it's crucial to make the best of it. This is challenging, but having a support system at home helps tremendously.*

*As I look back, I can understand and relate to some of these same actions in Dad, and empathize with how he may have felt as a teacher, a coach, a husband and a father of four. After seeing the help he's received from Dr. Gallagher, I'm so proud of him for overcoming all that he has. He's so much more relaxed, open-minded, and at ease—a happy place to be!*

From Jim's Son Jimmy:

*I never knew which father would be waiting for me when I came home at night or when I helped Dad in the yard or assisted him in coaching football. I was always on edge, waiting to see if he was in a good mood or angry and dealing with OCD thoughts—not knowing if I'd be praised or yelled at. By seven or eight, I understood when I could or couldn't interact with him. Oftentimes, I'd catch him standing in front of his dresser in his bedroom, staring in the mirror for long periods of time and talking to himself. I thought he was quietly praying, as he was making the sign of the cross, so I never interrupted him. He acted similarly in his coach's office at school between football practices and I could tell he was dealing with an OCD ritual because his lips were moving.*

*In elementary and middle school, I spent a great deal more time with Dad than my sisters did, going to football camps, practices, games and road trips during the season. Some of this was fun for me and some was hell. He coached me in junior high in basketball and baseball and always pushed me harder than my teammates to get better, but not in a bad way. He just wanted all of us to excel.*

From Jim's Middle Daughter Laura:

*As a child, my understanding of OCD was very limited and frankly skewed. I associated it with washing your hands repeatedly or going in and out of a room multiple times before actually entering. I never connected OCD with my dad in any way and I don't recall ever discussing it with anyone or relating it to our family. I attributed his behavior to his personality, demeanor, and the overall person he was. His temper, his getting lost in thought, his distance, and intensity—that was my father. It wasn't until adulthood that I was brought into the OCD conversation and exposed to what he'd been dealing with his entire life. I developed a better understanding of the depth of OCD, the intricacies of the disease, its effects, and the many different styles and symptoms it manifests. I realized that not only was my dad suffering, but as a child, I was, too.*

*While I make no assumptions or place blame, I believe that his OCD affected our ability to really be close and have a solid relationship. He was struggling within his own head and didn't have the time, patience or wherewithal to connect with his family the way he does now. Back then, he was often angry, short-tempered, and you didn't know which mood or Dad you'd get at any given time. Now I realize that he was constantly fighting his own internal demons, and I wish I'd known then what I do now. If our family had known, we'd* have helped him and been more patient and understanding, giving him the space and time he needed and deserved.

Since he's reached out to doctors and accepted help for what he couldn't control, I've seen a different side of him. He's much more compassionate, giving, happy and carefree. Our relationship, along with his relationship with his grandchildren, has flourished and is exceptional. For so long, he was caught up with something that doesn't just present itself as excessive hand washing and repetitiveness, but a silent illness with many other ramifications and challenges.

As my siblings and I have learned more about OCD, we realize that each of us suffers with it on different levels. Before having this recognition, I just assumed this was who I was. I use words like "particular, organized, picky, and focused" to describe myself, and some of that is accurate. But many times I let my head and my obsessiveness get the best of me—consumed by lists, placement of things, cleanliness and much more. I struggle with living in the moment and letting things go. I work daily to control this and remain a work in progress, trying to become the best version of myself.

As mental health issues have become more apparent and accepted in our culture, I hope that my dad's sharing his experience and journey—and his willingness to be so open and vulnerable—will shed light on OCD and allow other families to live with more compassion and love.

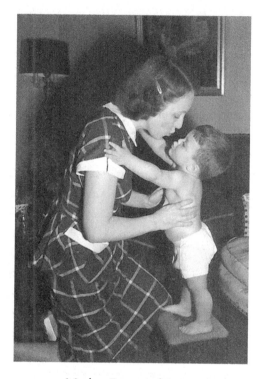

Mother Bette and Jamie
New York City, 1949

# Acknowledgments

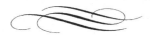

*I* would like to thank, first and foremost, Steve and Joyce Singular for sharing with me their vast knowledge and experience in writing and developing a book. Their suggestions, advice and counsel made this book possible. Thank you to my dear friends Paddy Burke, Brian King, Dave Higgins and Peter Appel for reading the manuscript and providing ideas, suggestions and corrections.

Thank you to Dr. David A. Lyons for being my primary mental health care physician for over 20 years, for prescribing medications and for recommending I consult with Dr. James Gallagher. Heartfelt thanks and appreciation goes to my good friend and confidant Jim Gallagher who changed my life for the better completely. Doc continues to provide for Betsy and me his professional expertise and experience in all matters pertaining to OCD and my therapy.

Sincere appreciation and thanks to my multi-talented cousin, John Cassano, for his time, effort and creativity in developing the front and back covers of this book.

And thank you to Gail Nelson, our graphic designer, who provided ongoing expertise in all areas related to completing and publishing the finished product.

Special thanks to our children, Amy, Laura, Jimmy and

Stephanie for taking the time and making the effort to contribute to this book by adding their thoughts. And most of all thank you to my best friend and wife Betsy. Betsy acted as primary typist, editor, writer and consultant on this manuscript. Betsy kept me centered and on task, and provided ongoing energy for the entire project. Without Betsy, there would be no book.

Made in the USA
Monee, IL
29 November 2019

17603021R10098